Meal Prep for Beginners

The Ultimate Guide to Weight Loss. Discover the Way to Burn Fat with Simple and Delicious Keto Recipes. Enjoy the 30 Days Intermittent Fasting Meal Plan.

Victoria Green

© **Copyright 2021 by Victoria Green- All rights reserved.**

ISBN: 978-1-914358-50-0

This document is geared towards providing exact and reliable information about the topic and issue covered. The publication is sold with the idea that the publisher is not required to render accounting, officially permitted, or otherwise qualified services. If advice is necessary, legal, or professional, a practiced individual in the profession should be ordered.

- From a Declaration of Principles which was accepted and approved equally by a Committee of the American Bar Association and a Committee of Publishers and Associations.

In no way is it legal to reproduce, duplicate, or transmit any part of this document in either electronic means or printed format. Recording of this publication is strictly prohibited, and any storage of this document is not allowed unless with written permission from the publisher. All rights reserved.

The information provided herein is stated to be truthful and consistent, in that any liability, in terms of inattention or otherwise, by any usage or abuse of any policies, processes, or directions contained within is the solitary and utter responsibility of the recipient reader. Under no circumstances will any legal responsibility or blame be held against the publisher for reparation, damages, or monetary loss due to the information herein, either directly or indirectly.

Respective authors own all copyrights not held by the publisher.

The information herein is offered for informational purposes solely and is universal as so. The presentation of the information is without a contract or any type of guarantee assurance.

The trademarks used are without any consent, and the publication of the trademark is without permission or backing by the trademark owner. All trademarks and brands within this book are for clarifying purposes only and are owned by the owners themselves, not affiliated with this document.

Table of Contents

PART 1

KETOGENIC DIET COOKBOOK FOR BEGINNERS	11
INTRODUCTION	12
MEAL PREP (RECIPES)	14
SNACKS AND APPETIZERS	14
1. KETO TACO CUPS	14
2. KETO SAUSAGE PUFFS	16
3. TA-KETOS	18
4. KETO BURGER WITH FAT BOMBS	19
5. PIZZA CHAFFLES	21
6. KETO TORTILLA CHIPS	23
7. ZUCCHINI TATER TOTS	24
8. BLT SUSHI	25
9. AVOCADO CHIPS	27
10. BUFFALO SHRIMP WITH LETTUCE WRAPS	28
11. KETO STUFFED PEPPERS	29
12. BACON-WRAPPED MOZZARELLA STICKS	31
13. NACHO CHEESE CRISPS	32
14. MAPLE BACON CARROTS	33
15. EGGPLANT PARM CHIPS	34
16. BACON ZUCCHINI FRIES	36
17. KETO QUESADILLAS	37
18. CREAMY AVOCADO DIP	39
19. BELL PEPPER NACHOS	39
20. PARM BOWLS	41

21. CHEESY CAULI BREAD ... 43

SOUPS AND STEWS ... 45

1. KETO BROCCOLI CHEDDAR ... 45
2. SPICY GINGER SCALLION ALONG WITH EGG DROP ZUCCHINI NOODLE ... 47
3. CHIPOTLE CHICKEN CHOWDER ... 48
4. KETO BACON CHEESEBURGER ... 51
5. SLOW-COOKER CHICKEN WITH CHILE VERDE ... 52
6. PALEO BEEF BRISKET PHO ... 55
7. 15-MINUTE GAZPACHO ALONG WITH CUCUMBER, RED PEPPER AND BASIL ... 59
8. GLUTEN-FREE MUSHROOM SOUP ... 60
9. INSTANT-POT BUFFALO CHICKEN SOUP ... 61
10. CREAMY AVOCADO CUCUMBER GAZPACHO ... 63
11. VEGAN CAULIFLOWER SOUP ... 64
12. CHICKEN ZUCCHINI NOODLE ... 66
13. INSTANT POT BUTTERNUT SQUASH ... 68
14. SLOW-COOKER CHICKEN FAJITA CHILI ... 70
15. CAULIFLOWER SOUP ALONG WITH COCONUT, TURMERIC AND LIME ... 72

SEAFOOD AND FISH ... 75

1. DILL SAUCE WITH TROUT OR SALMON ... 75
2. SALMON WITH A BACON TOMATO SAUCE ... 76
3. SKILLET SALMON WITH AN AVOCADO AND BASIL ... 79
4. KETO SALMON CAKES ... 82
5. TWO SALMON TARTARE ... 84
6. BAKED SALMON & ASPARAGUS IN FOIL ... 85
7. KETO SALMON & GLUTEN FREE TZATZIKI CUCUMBER NOODLES ... 87
8. SUPERB SALMON CEVICHE ... 89
9. ROASTED SALMON WITH A PARMESAN DILL CRUST ... 91
10. WALNUT (MAPLE) CRUSTED SALMON ... 92
11. SWEET CHILI SALMON ... 94

12. SALMON MEATBALLS WITH GARLIC LEMON CREAM SAUCE
 95
13. BAKED COD 97
14. PARMESAN BAKED COD 100
15. BUTTERED COD IN SKILLET 101
16. SIMPLE GARLIC SHRIMP ALFREDO WITH ZOODLES 102
17. KETO & PALEO PAD THAI WITH THE SHIRATAKI NOODLES
 104
18. LOBSTER TAILS WITH A GARLIC BUTTER 106
19. AVOCADO TUNA MELT 107
20. KETO TUNA CASSEROLE 109
21. GLUTEN FREE, LOW CARBOHYDRATE KETO CHIPS & FISH
 110
22. TUNA CAKES 112
23. KETO FISH PIE 115
24. SALMON IN A ROASTED PEPPER SAUCE 118
25. KETO FRIED FISH 120

VEGAN AND VEGETARIAN RECIPES 123

1. RATATOUILLE 123
2. WHOLE ROASTED CAULIFLOWER 125
3. BEST ARUGULA SALAD 127
4. ROASTED BRUSSELS SPROUTS 127
5. INSTANT - POT VEGETABLE SOUP 129
6. EASIEST-EVER GUACAMOLE 131
7. ZUCCHINI CAULIFLOWER FRITTERS 132
8. ZUCCHINI NOODLES WITH AN AVOCADO SAUCE 134
9. AVOCADO CHOCOLATE MOUSSE 135
11. LOW CARBOHYDRATE CINNAMON MUG ROLL CAKE 138
12. CARROT CAKE BITES 140
13. MEXICAN-CHOCOLATE AVOCADO ICE CREAM 142
14. KETO BROCCOLI SALAD 144
15. ALMOND FLOUR WAFFLES 145
16. EVERYTHING KETO BAGELS 147
17. ARTICHOKE STUFFED PEPPERS 149
18. BEST KETO TORTILLAS 150
19. ZUCCHINI GRILLED CHEESE 153

20. Bell Pepper Nachos 154
21. Cheesy Cauli Bread 156
22. Easy Keto Cere 158
23. Baked-Egg Av(ado Boats 160
24. Cauliflower `)ast 161

SALADS 163

1. Keto Egg S/ .ad 163
2. Grilled Ch cken Salad 164
3. Cobb Egg alad 166
4. Loaded C auliflower Salad 167
5. Shrimp(de Gallo 168
6. Chicken Salad Stuffed Avocados 170
7. Parmesan Brussels Sprouts Salad 171
8. Shrimp Salad 173
9. Antipasto Salad 174
10. Greek Salad 176
11. Strawberry Spinach Salad 177
12. Caprese Salad 178
13. Arugula Salad 179
14. Grilled Chicken Wedge Salad 180
15. Cilantro-Lime Cucumber Salad 182
16. Greek Salmon Salad with Tahini Yogurt Dressing
    183

SMOOTHIES 187

1. Triple berry avocado 187
2. Chocolate Peanut (Butter) 188
3. Strawberry zucchini chia 189
4. Coconut blackberry mint 189
5. Lemon cucumber green smoothie 190
6. Cinnamon raspberry breakfast smoothie 190
7. Strawberries and cream smoothie 191
8. Chocolate cauliflower breakfast smoothie 192
9. Pumpkin spice smoothie 192

10. Lime pie smoothie   193

DESSERTS   194

1. Keto Sugar-Free Cheesecake   194
2. Keto Chocolate Chip Cookies   196
3. Keto Chocolate Cake   197
4. Keto Chocolate Mug Cake   200
5. Keto Ice Cream   201
6. Keto Hot Chocolate   202
7. Keto Pumpkin Cheesecake   203
8. Keto Pumpkin Pie   206
9. Keto Peanut Butter Cookies   208
10. Magic Keto Cookies   209
11. Chocolate Keto Cookies   210
12. Keto Walnut Snowballs   212
13. Keto Pecan Crescents   214
14. Keto Frosty   216
15. Keto Peanut Butter Sandies   217
16. Keto Brownies   218
17. Chocolate Keto Protein Shake   220
18. Keto Double Chocolate Muffins   221
19. Cookie Dough Keto Fat Bombs   222
20. Keto Avocado Pops   223
21. Keto Chocolate Truffles   224
22. Carrot Cake Keto Balls   225
23. Chocolate Blueberry Clusters   226
24. Keto Fat Bombs   227
25. Chocolate Covered Strawberry Cubes   229
26. Keto Brownie Bombs   229
27. Sugar-Free Low Carb Keto Avocado Brownies   230
29. Keto Peanut Butter Cheesecake Bites   233
30. Paleo Vegan Coconut Crack Bars - Healthy 3 Ingredient - No Bake   234
31. Healthy Minute Low Carb Cinnamon Roll Mug Cake   235
32. Homemade Sugar-Free Nutella   237

CONCLUSION	239

PART 2

INTERMITTENT FASTING	241
INTRODUCTION	242
CHAPTER 1: RECIPES FOR FASTING DIET	248
BERRY PARFAIT	249
ROASTED CAULIFLOWER RICE	250
BULLETPROOF COFFEE	252
MUSTARD GREEN BEANS	253
ESSENTIAL BONE BROTH	255
HOMEMADE CHICKEN FINGERS	257
GRAIN-FREE PANCAKES	260
STEAK FAJITAS	262
MINI FRITTATAS	265
ARUGULA AND PROSCIUTTO SALAD	267
SIMPLE HOMEMADE BACON	268
PEAR AND ARUGULA SALAD WITH PINE NUTS	271
GRAIN-FREE CAULIFLOWER PIZZA	273
STRAWBERRY AND KALE SALAD	274
CHICKEN "BREADED" IN PORK RINDS	275
TOMATO, CUCUMBER, AND AVOCADO SALAD	277
CHICKEN DRUMSTICKS WRAPPED IN BACON	279
AVOCADO FRIES	280
CHICKEN STUFFED BELL PEPPERS	283
GAME DAY WINGS	285

CHAPTER 2: INTERMITTENT KETO RECIPES 288

Pecan & Coconut 'N' Oatmeal	289
Boiled Eggs with Spiced Asparagus Soldiers	290
Bacon, Egg & Cheese Breakfast "Muffins"	292
Easy Bacon and Egg Muffins	294
Cheddar Chive Baked Avocado Eggs	295
Baked Salmon and Eggs with Chives	297
Blueberry Almond Pancakes	299
Porridge with Pistachios and Chia	301
Speedy Eggs and Avocado	303
Berry Breakfast Shake	304
Cheddar, Spinach & Mushroom Omelet	305
6. Now fold the plain side of the egg over the veges half to make a half-moon. Cook for another 1 minute. Serve straight away.	307
Tomato and Basil Omelette	308
Bacon, Avocado & Turkey Lettuce Wraps	310
Hummus in a Hurry	311
Spicy Sesame Zoodles	313
Tapenade with Feta	315
Italian Stuffed Peppers	316
Warm Spinach & Roast Chicken Salad With Bacon Vinaigrette	319
Spanish Aubergine Stew with Chorizo	321
Kimchi Pork Lettuce Cups	323
Balsamic Fried Pork Steak with Garlicky White Bean Mash	325

CHAPTER 3: STARTING IF YOUR FIRST 30 DAYS 328

3.1   Intermittent fasting tips & tricks   333

GLOSSARY 337

CONCLUSION 340

PART 1

Ketogenic Diet Cookbook for Beginners

Introduction

Low-carb diets were falling in and out of fashion long before the Atkins days. Yet a far more stringent type of low carbohydrate eating, recognized as the ketogenic diet, is now drawing media attention, triggering a fierce medical discussion over its perceived risks and benefits.

Ketogenic diets and Atkins frequently encourage followers to free sugars from their items. So, while the Atkins diet steadily decreases calories over time, Keto imposes stringent limits on carbs and protein. The carbohydrate system is weakened from this form of feeding, forcing it to absorb fat and generate an extra energy source called ketones. A conventional ketogenic diet reduces carbohydrates to less than 10% of calories and 20% of protein, whereas the remainder is fat.

In best-selling novels, promoted by celebrities, and admired as an antidote to numerous illnesses, the keto diet is now famous. Proponents say that it encourages dramatic weight reduction and may dramatically improve their blood sugar concentrations for type II diabetes, decreasing when individuals miss carbs.

Numerous ketogenic diet trials have been performed throughout the years, but most were minimal and very short. A federal Clinical Study suggests more than 70 current or early trials exploring the effect of diet on cognitive, cardiovascular, and metabolic well-being.

The ketogenic diet, and there is a reason, has become so common. It's working and losing weight is just a start. Analysis has found a stabilizing mental condition. It raises energy prices as well as controlling blood sugar. It decreases blood pressure, raises potassium, and many have personally seen the outcomes of their lives. The bulk of people spend years consuming unhealthy food in their teens and early 20s. Today, existence is dominated by packaged and refined food containing tonnes of sugar, low energy, fear, and depression. Many citizens feel frightened by Keto. They don't have to eat them for a decent sum of income. Maybe they're scared their favorite meal will be lost.

Meal Prep (Recipes)
Snacks and appetizers

1. Keto Taco Cups

Yields: 1 Dozen servings | Prep Time: 10 Mins | Total time: 30 Mins

Ingredients

- Shredded cheddar 2 cup
- Extra-virgin olive oil 1 tbsp.
- Onion, chopped, 1 small
- Garlic, minced, 3 cloves
- Ground beef 1 lb.

- Chili powder 1 tsp.
- Ground cumin 1/2 tsp.
- Paprika 1/2 tsp.
- Kosher salt
- Ground black pepper
- Sour cream
- Diced avocado
- Sliced tomatoes
- Sliced cilantro

Directions

1. Preheat the oven to 375°c and cover the wide baking sheet with parchment paper. Add approximately 2 teaspoons of cheddar a couple of inches away. Bake until the bulb and the edges start to turn golden, around 6 minutes. Let it cool down on the baking sheet for a minute.

2. In the meantime, oil the bottom of the muffin tin with a cooking spray, then gently pick up the melting cheese slices and put them on the bottom of the muffin tin. Pair along with another inverted muffin tin and let it cool for 9-10

minutes. If you don't have a separate muffin box, use hands to help form the cheese inside the inverted muffin tin.

3. Heat oil in a large skillet over medium heat. Add the onion and fry, stirring regularly, until softened, for around 5 minutes. Stir in the garlic, then add the ground beef, dissolve the meat with a spoon. Cook until beef is not yellow, around 6 minutes, then remove the grease.

4. Return the meat to the stew and season with chili powder, paprika, cumin, salt, and pepper.

5. Move the cheese cups to the serving tray. Cover with boiled ground beef and finish with avocado, sour cream, cilantro, and tomatoes.

2. Keto Sausage Puffs

Yields: 3 Dozen servings | Prep Time: 10 Mins | Total Time: 50 Mins

Ingredients

- Olive oil 1 tbsp.
- Italian sausage 1 lb.
- Shredded cheddar, divided, 1 c.

- Cream cheese 2 oz.

- Grated parmesan 2 tbsp.

- Egg 1 large

- Almond flour 1 c.

- Baking powder 1 tsp.

- Kosher salt 1/2 tsp.

Directions

1. Preheat the oven to 400°C and cover the baking sheet with parchment paper.

2. Heat oil in a large skillet over medium-high heat. Add the sausage and cook. Dissolve the meat with a spoon, till golden, around 7 minutes. Remove from the heat.

3. In a medium, microwave-safe dish, melt 1/4 cup cheddar, cream cheese, and parmesan cheese. Add the cooked sausages, egg, baking powder, almond flour, and salt and mix to blend. Mix in the surplus 3/4 cup of cheddar.

4. Using a small cookie scoop, shape a mixture of 1" balls and put on the prepared baking sheet. Bake until the sausage is cooked through and golden for 20 to 22 minutes.

3. Ta-Ketos

Yields: 1 Dozen servings | Prep Time: 15 Mins | Total time: 45 Mins

Ingredients

- Olive oil 2 tbsp.
- Onion, finely chopped, 1/2
- Garlic, minced, 4 cloves
- Ground cumin 1 tsp.
- Chili powder 1 tsp.
- Shredded chicken 2 c.
- Red enchilada sauce 2/3 c.
- Freshly chopped cilantro 4 tbsp.
- Kosher salt
- Shredded cheddar 2 cup
- Shredded Monterey jack 2 cup
- Sour cream (optional)

Directions

1. Set the oven to 375°C, preheat it and line two baking papers with parchment paper. Heat oil in a medium skillet over medium heat. Add the

onion and cook until tender, 3 minutes. Add garlic and spices and simmer for 1 to 2 minutes, until fragrant. Remove the chicken and the enchilada sauce and get the mixture to a boil. Stir in coriander, season with salt, and remove from the heat.

2. Create taquito shells: blend cheeses in a medium dish. Divide the mixture into twelve 3 1/2" piles on the prepared baking sheet. Bake until the cheese is molten and mildly golden around the edges, around 10 minutes. Let it cool for 2 to 5 minutes, then remove the shells off the parchment. Add a little pile of chicken and roll firmly. Repeat again and again until all the taquitos are prepared.

3. Marinade with cilantro and serve along with sour cream.

4. Keto Burger with Fat Bombs

Yields: 20 servings | Prep. Time: 15 Mins | Tot. Time: 30 Mins

Ingredients

- Ground beef 1 lb.
- Garlic powder 1/2 tsp.
- Kosher salt
- Cooking spray
- Ground black pepper
- Cold butter, cut into 20 pieces, 2 tbsp.
- Cheddar, cut into 20 pieces, 2 oz.
- Lettuce leaves, for serving
- Thinly chopped tomatoes, for serving
- Mustard, for serving

Directions

1. Preheat the oven to 375°C and grease the mini muffin tin with a cooking spray. Season beef with garlic powder, salt, and pepper in a medium dish.

2. Add 1 teaspoon of beef uniformly to the bottom of each muffin tin cup, covering the bottom entirely. Place a slice of butter on top, then add 1 teaspoon of beef over the butter to cover it entirely.

3. Put a slice of cheddar on top of the meat in each cup, press the remaining beef over the cheese to cover it entirely.

4. Bake for about 15 minutes before the meat is cooked through. Let it cool a bit.

5. Properly use a metal offset spatula to remove each burger from the tin. Serve with cabbage, tomatoes, and mustard.

5. Pizza Chaffles

Yields: 2 servings | Prep Time: 5 Mins | Total Time: 15 Mins

Ingredients

For Pizza Chaffles:

- Eggs 2 large
- Almond flour 2 tbsp.
- Baking soda 1/2 tsp.
- Kosher salt 1/2 tsp.
- Shredded mozzarella 1 1/2 c.
- Pepperoni slices 1/3 c.
- Grated Parmesan

Directions

1. Preheat the waffle maker (follow the manufacturer's instructions). In a medium bowl, stir together eggs, salt, almond flour, and soda. Add 1 cup of mozzarella and whisk to coat.

2. Add 1/2 cup of the mixture to the waffle maker's center and cook till golden and crisp, 2 to 3 minutes. Repeat the residual batter.

3. Instantly top with marinara, remaining 1/2 cup mozzarella, pepperoni, and a sprinkle of parmesan cheese.

6. Keto Tortilla Chips

Yield: 4-5 servings | Prep Time: 5 Mins | Total Time: 30-35 Mins

Ingredients

- Shredded mozzarella 2 c.
- Almond flour 1 c.
- Kosher salt 1 tsp.
- Garlic powder 1 tsp.
- Chili powder 1/2 tsp.
- Ground black pepper

Directions

1. Preheat the oven to 350°C. Line two large baking sheets of parchment paper.

2. Melt mozzarella in a microwave-safe bowl, about 1 minute and 30 seconds. Add almond flour, garlic powder, salt, chili powder and a few cracks of black pepper. Knead the dough a few times using your hands until the ball is smooth.

3. Place the dough among two sheets of parchment paper and flip into a rectangle 1/8" thick. Cut the dough into triangles using pizza cutter or a knife.

4. Spread the chips on the prepared baking sheets and cook until the edges are golden and begin to be crisp, 12 to 14 minutes.

7. Zucchini Tater Tots

Servings: 4 | Prep Time: 10 Mins | Total Time: 30 Mins

Ingredients

- Zucchini, grated (about 5 c.) 3 mediums
- Eggs, lightly beaten, 2 larges
- Shredded cheddar 1/2 c.
- Grated parmesan 1/2 c.
- Dried oregano 1 tsp.
- Garlic powder 1/4 tsp.
- Kosher salt
- Ground black pepper
- Ketchup, for serving

Directions

1. Preheat the oven to 400°C and oil the baking sheet with a cooking spray. Put the zucchini in the kitchen towel and drain any excess liquid.

2. In a big dish, add zucchini, salt, egg, parmesan, cheddar, oregano, garlic powder, and pepper. Take about 1 tablespoon of the mixture and roll it into a pattern form with your fingertips and place on a baking sheet. Cook for 15-20 minutes or until golden. Serve the ketchup.

8. BLT Sushi

Yields: 2 servings | Prep Time: 10 Mins | Total Time: 45 Mins

Ingredients

- Bacon 10 slices
- Mayonnaise 2 tbsp.
- Tomatoes 1 c. Chopped
- Avocado, diced, 1/2

- Shredded romaine 1 c.
- Kosher salt
- Ground black pepper

Directions

1. Preheat the oven to 400°C and put a wire rack over a wide baking sheet. Place 5 slices of bacon side by side. Lift one end of each slice of bacon and put another slice of bacon on top of the raised pieces. Put the slices inside. Then, raise back the slices of bacon opposite and put a slice of bacon on top. Place the slices back down. Repeat the weaving method until you have a weave of 5 strips of bacon in 5 strips. Set the bacon weave to the prepared baking sheet.

2. Bake until the bacon is fried but always foldable for 20 mins.

3. Pat bacon weave with paper towels to remove fat and move to a plastic wrap sheet (it helps to roll).

4. Spread the mayonnaise on top of the bacon in a thin layer, then the top-bottom third of the bacon weave with tomatoes and avocado. Sprinkle with romaine and add salt and pepper.

5. Starting from the rim, roll closely, then cut crosswise into "sushi rolls."

9. Avocado Chips

Yields: 15 servings | Prep Time: 5 Mins | Total Time: 40 Mins

Ingredients

- Ripe avocado 1 large
- Freshly grated parmesan 3/4 c.
- Lemon juice 1 tsp.
- Garlic powder 1/2 tsp.
- Italian seasoning 1/2 tsp.
- Kosher salt
- Ground black pepper

Directions

1. Preheat the oven to 325°C and cover two baking sheets with parchment paper. In a medium dish, mash the avocado with a fork until it is smooth. Stir in Parmesan, garlic powder, lemon juice, and Italian seasonings. Season to taste with salt and pepper.

2. Place teaspoon-size mixture scoops on a baking sheet, leaving around 3" apart across each scoop. Flatten each scoop to 3" wide with a back of a spoon or a measuring cup. Bake till crisp and golden, about 30 minutes, then let it cool entirely. Serve at room temperature.

10. Buffalo Shrimp with Lettuce Wraps

Servings: 4 | Prep Time: 15 Mins | Tot Time: 35 Mins

Ingredients

- Butter 1/4 tbsp.
- Garlic, minced, 2 cloves
- Hot sauce, such as Frank's, 1/4 c.
- Olive oil 1 tbsp.
- Shrimp, peeled, tails removed, 1 lb.
- Kosher salt
- Romaine, leaves separated, 1 head
- Onion, finely chopped, 1/4 red
- Rib celery, sliced thin, 1
- Blue cheese, crumbled, 1/2 c.

Directions

1. Made buffalo sauce: Melt butter in a small saucepan over medium heat. Add the garlic and cook till fragrant, 1 minute. Add the hot sauce and mix until combined. Switch the fire to low when you're frying shrimp.

2. Create shrimp: heat oil in a large skillet over medium heat. Add shrimp and dress with salt and pepper to taste. Cook, turning halfway, until pink and opaque on all sides, around 2 minutes per hand. Switch off the heat and add the buffalo sauce to the coat.

3. Assemble wraps: add a little scoop of shrimp to the middle of the Roman leaf, then finish with red onion, celery, and blue cheese.

11. Keto Stuffed Peppers

Servings: 8 | Prep Time: 15 Mins | Tot Time: 1 hour 15 mins

Ingredients

- Bacon, cut into 1/2" strips, 4 slices
- Onion, chopped, 1/2 medium

- Ground beef 1 lb.
- Chili powder 1 tbsp.
- Ground cumin 2 tsp.
- Dried oregano 1 tsp.
- Paprika 1 tsp.
- Kosher salt
- Ground black pepper
- Beef broth 1 c. Low-sodium
- Diced tomatoes, drained, 1 (14.5-oz.) Can
- Bell peppers, sliced in half, 4
- Shredded cheddar 2 c.
- Thinly chopped green onions 2 tbsp.

Directions

1. Preheat the oven to 350°C. In a big pot over medium heat, integrate bacon and cook for 8 minutes until crispy. Drain on a paper towel-lined pan.
2. Add the onion to the pot and simmer for 5 minutes until tender. Add beef and prepare. Dissolve the meat with a wooden spoon until it is no longer yellow, 7 minutes. Add chili powder,

oregano, cumin, and pepper. Season to taste with salt and pepper.

3. Add the butter and tomatoes and put them to a simmer. Reduce heat and boil until lightly thickened for 20 minutes.

4. Put the bell pepper half in a broad baking dish and cover with chili. Cover with cheddar and bacon and simmer until the cheese has melted and the peppers are softened for about 30 minutes.

5. Until eating, garnish with green onions.

12. Bacon-Wrapped Mozzarella Sticks

Yields: 1 Dozen servings | Prep Time: 5 Mins | Total Time: 2 hours 45 mins

Ingredients

- String cheese 12 sticks
- Bacon 12 slices
- Italian seasoning 2 tsp.
- Marinara, for serving

Directions

1. Unwrap the cheese and put it on a plate or a small baking sheet. Freeze until strong, 4 hours until overnight.

2. Preheat the oven to 400°C and cover the medium baking sheet with foil. Place the bacon with an even layer and sprinkle with the Italian seasonings. Bake until mildly crisp but always folding, for 12 to 15 minutes.

3. Take the bacon from the oven and let it cool slowly. Line up a small baking sheet with foil.

4. Cover 1 strip of bacon in each frozen stick of string cheese. Put on the covered baking sheet and cook until the bacon is crisp, and the cheese is only beginning to melt, 5 - 8 minutes.

5. Serve with marinara on the edge of the dip.

13. Nacho Cheese Crisps

Yields: 6 servings | Prep Time: 5 Mins | Total Time: 55 Mins

Ingredients

- Sliced cheddar 1 (8-oz.) Package

- Taco seasoning 2 tsp.

Directions

1. Preheat the oven to 250°C and line a large baking sheet of parchment paper. Break each cheese slice into 9 squares and put it in a medium dish. Add the taco seasoning and toss the coat.

2. Place cheese slices in an even layer (make sure nothing is overlapping) on a lined baking dish. Bake for 40 minutes until crisp and golden (they will crisp up even more when cooled). Let it cool for 10 minutes, then extract from the parchment paper.

14. Maple Bacon Carrots

Yields: 12 servings | Prep Time: 5 Mins | Total Time 35 Mins

Ingredients

- Carrots, peeled, 12 mediums
- Bacon 12 strips
- Maple syrup 1/4
- Ground black pepper

Directions

1. Preheat the oven to 400°C. Wrap each carrot in one rasher of bacon and put the bacon on a wide baking sheet. Rub with maple syrup all over and season with black pepper.

2. Bake for 10 minutes, take from the oven and brush with the remaining maple syrup. Bake for 15 minutes, until the carrots are tender and the bacon is crisp. Serve it.

15. Eggplant Parm Chips

Yields: 4 servings | Prep Time: 5 Mins | Total Time: 50 Mins

Ingredients

- Eggplant 1 medium
- Kosher salt

- Olive oil 2 tbsp.

- Freshly grated Parmesan 1/4 c.

- Italian seasoning 1 tsp.

- Garlic powder 1 tsp.

- Ground black pepper

- Marinara, for dipping (optional)

Directions

1. Preheat the oven to 350°C. Break the eggplant into very thin layer rounds—on the mandolin, if necessary. Then place on the paper towels the eggplant slices in a thin and even layer. Season gently with salt, and let it rest for 10 minutes. Wipe some noticeable moisture away from the slices along with a paper towel and flip it. Repeat the steps.

2. Move the eggplant slices to the wide bowl and discard them in the liquid. Add Parmesan, Italian seasonings, and garlic powder. Sprinkle with black pepper and stir until the slices are finely covered.

3. Arrange the eggplant slices in an even layer (make sure nothing is overlapping) on a broad baking sheet.

4. Bake until golden and dry, for 16 to 18 minutes. Let it cool before serving with marinara.

16. Bacon Zucchini Fries

Servings: 8 | Prep Time: 10 Mins | Tot Time: 50 Mins

Ingredients

- Cooking spray
- Zucchini, cut into wedges, 4
- Bacon 16 strips
- Ranch, for serving

Directions

1. Preheat the oven to 425°C and coat a baking sheet with a cooking spray. Cover each wedge of zucchini in bacon and put it on a baking sheet.

2. Bake till the bacon is cooked through it and crisp, around 35 minutes. Serve the ranch.

17. Keto Quesadillas

Servings: 4 | Prep Time: 10 Mins | Tot Time: 35 Mins

Ingredients

- Olive oil 1 tbsp.
- Bell pepper, sliced, 1
- Onion, sliced, 1/2 yellow
- Chili powder 1/2 tsp.
- Kosher salt
- Ground black pepper
- Shredded Monterey Jack 3 c.
- Shredded cheddar 3 c.
- Shredded chicken 4 c.
- Avocado, thinly sliced, 1
- Onion, thinly sliced, 1 green
- Sour cream, for serving

Directions

1. Preheat the oven to 400°C and line two medium-sized baking sheets with parchment paper.

2. Heat oil in a medium saucepan over medium heat. Add pepper and onion and season to taste with chili powder, salt, and pepper. Cook until tender, for 5 minutes. Move it to a tray.

3. In a medium dish, whisk the cheeses together. In the middle of the two prepared baking sheets, add 1 1/2 cups of cheese mixture. Spread into an even layer and build a circle, the shape of a flour tortilla.

4. Bake the cheese until it is melted and mildly golden across the outside, for 8 to 10 minutes. Add the onion-pepper blend, the shredded chicken, and the avocado slices to half of each. Let cool slowly, then use the parchment paper and a tiny spatula to carefully raise and fold one side of the "tortilla" cheese over the part with the fillings. Return to the oven for 3 to 4 minutes. Repeat to produce two more quesadillas.

5. Break the quesadilla into pieces. Until eating, garnish with green onion and sour cream.

18. Creamy Avocado Dip

Yields: 4 servings | Prep Time: 5 Mins | Total Time: 5 Mins

Ingredients

- Avocados 2 ripe
- Plain Greek yogurt 1/2 c.
- Garlic, minced 2 cloves
- Juice of 1 lime
- Ground black pepper
- Kosher salt

Directions

1. In a bowl place the avocados and crush them with a fork.
2. Stir in yogurt, lime juice, garlic, and season well with salt and pepper.
3. Serve with a few chips and veggies.

19. Bell Pepper Nachos

Yields: 6 servings | Prep Time: 15 Mins | Total Time: 40 Mins

Ingredients

- Bell peppers 4
- Olive oil 2 tbsp.
- Ground cumin 1/2 tsp.
- Chili powder 1/2 tsp.
- Garlic powder 1/4 tsp.
- Kosher salt
- Ground black pepper
- Shredded Monterey jack 1 1/2 cup
- Guacamole 1 c.
- Pickled jalapeño slices 1/2 cup
- Shredded cheddar 1 1/2 cup
- Sour cream 1/2 cup
- Milk (or water) 1 tbsp.
- Pico de Gallo salsa 1 cup
- Lime wedges, for serving

Directions

1. Preheat the oven to 425°C and cover two narrow baking sheets with foil.

2. Divide the bell peppers onto the baking sheets. Stir in olive oil, cumin, chili powder and garlic powder. Season with salt and pepper generously. Bake until the peppers are crisp, around 10 minutes.

3. Top bell peppers with cheddar and Monterey Jack. Bake until cheese is bubbly, around ten minutes.

4. Cover with guacamole, sauce, and jalapeños. In a shallow dish, mix the sour cream and milk and drizzle over the bell peppers. Squeeze the lime wedge at the end and serve with more lime wedges.

20. Parm Bowls

Yields: 8 servings | Prep Time: 5 Mins | Total Time: 25 Mins

Ingredients

- Shredded Parmesan 2 cups
- Cooking spray

Directions

1. Preheat the oven to 375°C. Line a large baking sheet of parchment paper and mist well with a cooking spray. Create a tablespoon of Parmesan and cook until melty, 5 minutes.

2. Using a spatula or your fingertips to raise a pile of cheese and position it over a 4" diameter upside-down cup, softly pushing to mould it across the bowl. Repeat for the remaining cheese.

3. Let the Parm shells cool until they are hardened, then gently extract from the bowls. Fill with Caesar salad or toppings.

21. Cheesy Cauli Bread

Yields: 1 dozen servings | Prep Time: 5 Mins | Total Time: 45 Mins

Ingredients

- Head cauliflower 1 large
- Eggs 2 large
- Garlic, minced, 2 cloves
- Dried oregano 1/2 tsp.
- Shredded mozzarella, divided, 3 c.
- Grated parmesan 1/2 c.
- Kosher salt
- Ground black pepper
- Pinch of red pepper
- Freshly chopped parsley 2 tsp.
- Marinara, for dipping

Directions

1. Preheat the oven to 425°C and line the parchment baking sheet. Cauliflower grate on a rack or in a food processor.

2. Move the cauliflower to a large bowl of eggs, basil, oregano, 1 cup of parmesan, mozzarella, and season with salt and pepper. Stir before the combination is fully mixed.

3. Take the dough and move it to the prepared baking sheet and pat it to the crust. Bake for 25 minutes, until golden and crisp.

4. Sprinkle with the leftover mozzarella, crushed chili flakes and parsley and simmer until cheese is melted for 5 to 10 minutes.

5. Cut it and eat it.

Soups and stews

1. Keto Broccoli Cheddar

Servings: 4 | Prep Time: 20 Mins | Tot Time: 20 Mins

Ingredients

- Butter 2 tablespoons
- White Onion 1/ 8 Cup
- Garlic, finely minced, 1/2 teaspoon
- Chicken Broth 2 Cups
- Salt and Pepper, to taste
- Broccoli, chopped, 1 Cup
- Cream Cheese 1 Tablespoon

- Heavy Whipping Cream 1/4 Cup
- Cheddar Cheese; shredded, 1 Cup
- Bacon; Cooked and Crumbled (Optional), 2 Slices
- Xanthan gum (optional, for thickening), 1/2 teaspoon

Directions

1. In a big pot, sauté the onion and garlic with butter on medium heat until the onions are softened and translucent.
2. Add the broth and the broccoli to the pot and cook the broccoli until soft. Add salt, pepper, and seasoning.
3. Put the cream cheese in a small bowl and heat in a microwave for ~30 seconds until soft and simple to stir.
4. Stir in the broth strong whipped cream and cream cheese; carry to a simmer.
5. Turn the heat off and whisk easily in cheddar cheese.
6. Serve hot with crumbs of bacon (optional)

2. Spicy Ginger Scallion along with Egg Drop Zucchini Noodle

Yields: 2 servings | Prep Time: 10 Mins | Total Time: 25 Mins

Ingredients

- Olive oil 1 tablespoon
- Scallions, sliced, 1 bunch
- Garlic clove 1 large
- Red pepper flakes 1/4-1/2 teaspoon
- Minced ginger 1.5 tablespoons
- Sherry vinegar 1 tablespoon
- Soy sauce, low sodium, 2 tablespoons
- Vegetable broth 4 cups
- Water 1 cup
- Eggs, beaten, 2 mediums
- Zucchini, bladed, 1 medium
- Ground black pepper

Directions

1. In a wide saucepan put the oli and heat it over medium-high heat. After the oil has shimmered,

add the white sections of the scallions, garlic, red pepper flakes, ginger, and simmer for 3 minutes or until the scallions begin to soften.

2. Add the sherry vinegar, soya sauce, vegetable broth and water. Get things to a simmer.

3. When the broth is boiling, reduce to mild and gently add in the egg while swirling the broth to render the egg wisps.

4. Put the remaining green pieces of the scallions in the zucchini noodles and cook for 2-3 minutes until the zucchini is softened to al dente. Divide the broth into two cups, season with black pepper and eat.

3. Chipotle Chicken Chowder

Yield: 6-8 servings | Prep Time: 15 Mins | Total Time: 1 hour

Ingredients

- Butter 2 tbsp.
- Onion, diced, ½ of a yellow
- Pepper, diced, ½ of a red

- Garlic, minced, 4 cloves
- Salt 1 tsp.
- Black pepper ½ tsp.
- Cumin 1 tsp.
- Dried oregano ¼ tsp.
- Dried thyme ¼ tsp.
- All-purpose flour 2 tbsp.
- Whole milk 1½ c.
- Chicken broth 4 c. Or (1) 32 oz. Box
- Chipotle chile in adobo, 1
- Adobo sauce (from chipotle chilies) 2 tsp.
- Hatch chilies ½ (4 oz.) Can
- Fire-roasted diced tomatoes ½ (14.5 oz.) Can
- Size red potatoes 5 medium
- Corn 2 c. Fresh or frozen
- Diced chicken, 2 c. Cooked
- Cheddar cheese, grated, 1 c. Medium-sharp
- Garnishes
- Grated cheddar cheese

- Chopped cilantro
- Lime wedges

Directions

1. Melt the butter in a big Dutch oven or stockpot over medium heat. Add the onion and the red pepper, sauté until soft and add the garlic. When the garlic is fragrant and transparent, sprinkle with the flour with the seasonings (salt, cumin, pepper, oregano, and thyme). Cook for 1-2 minutes or until the flour is softly golden-colored (but not brown). Whisk in a broth of milk and chicken. Remove chipotle chilies, hot peppers, adobo sauce, and roasted tomatoes. Get things to a simmer.

2. When the mixture is boiling, add the potatoes and the corn, decrease to medium heat once. Boil until the potatoes are fork-tender, around 15 to 20 minutes. Stir in the minced chicken and cheese and stir until the cheese is fully melted. Continue cooking for another 15 minutes. Garnish with lime, cilantro, and cheese.

4. Keto Bacon Cheeseburger

Yields: 2 servings | Prep Time: 5 Mins | Total Time: 20 Mins

Ingredients

- Lean ground beef 1 pound
- Onion ½ medium
- Fire-roasted tomatoes ½ can
- Beef broth 3 cups
- Bacon ¼ cup cooked
- Chopped pickle jalapeno 1 tablespoon
- Salt 1 teaspoon
- Pepper ½ teaspoon
- Garlic powder ½ teaspoon
- Worcestershire sauce 2 teaspoons
- Cream cheese 4 ounces
- Shredded cheddar cheese 1 cup
- Pickle spear 1

Directions

1. Click the Sauté button and add beef to the ground. Brown beef midway adds the onion. Continue cooking beef once there is no pink remaining. Click the Cancel tab, please. Add onions, broth, bacon, salt, jalapenos, pepper, garlic, and Worcestershire sauce and stir. In the center, put the cream cheese on top.

2. Tap on the lid closed. Click the Soup button to change the time for 15 minutes. When the timer beeps, relieve the pressure easily. Cover with sliced pickles and marinade with shredded cheddar.

5. Slow-Cooker Chicken with Chile Verde

Yields: 6 servings | Prep time: 1 hour | Total Time: 8 hours

Ingredients

- Tomatillos 2 pounds
- Poblano or Anaheim peppers 4
- Jalapeños 2-3
- Garlic 2-3 cloves

- Diced green chiles 1 - 4 oz can
- Cilantro 1 bunch
- Juice of 1 lime
- Ground cumin 2 teaspoons
- Dried oregano 2 teaspoons
- Salt 1/4 teaspoon
- Ground black pepper
- Low-sodium, chicken broth 3/4 cup
- Boneless and Skinless Chicken Thighs 2 pounds
- Yellow onion, diced, 1 large

Directions

1. Place the cut-sided tomatillos, jalapeños, poblano peppers, and non-peeled cloves of garlic on a large foil-lined baking sheet. If necessary, use two baking sheets. Cook under the broiler until the tomatillos and peppers tend to roast and blacken (about 8-10 minutes). If you don't have a broiler in your oven, you should set the oven at 425 degrees F (this option may take longer).

2. Move the poblano and jalapeno peppers to a plastic Ziploc bag and zip it securely. It's all right if you don't extract the skin completely—the most critical component is eliminating the seeds and roots.

3. While the peppers are steaming in the bag, add the tomatoes to the blender. Peel the garlic cloves and add the peppers, green chilies, cilantro, lime juice, oregano, cumin, salt, pepper, and chicken broth to the blender. Mix the components so they are well mixed.

4. Add the chicken thighs and the sliced onions to the slow cooker, pour the tomatillo-chile sauce over the chicken's top, and mix to blend. Cover and cook on the upper part for 3 hours or in the lower part for 7 hours.

5. Until eating, remove the chicken with a slotted spoon and break it with a fork. Add back to the slow cooker and mix with a spoon. Taste and change the seasoning as required. Serve with brown rice, corn tortilla, tortilla chips and/or beans.

6. Paleo Beef Brisket Pho

Servings: 8 | Prep Time: 20 Mins | Tot Time: 1 hour

Ingredients

- Beef brisket 1.75 - 2 lbs.
- Beef shank soup bones 1-1.25 lbs.
- Shiitake mushrooms 1 ¼ cups dry
- Carrots, roughly chopped, 3 loose
- Yellow onion, peeled, 1 medium size
- Leek 1 large size
- Water
- Fine sea salt 2 ½ tsp

- Red Boat fish sauce 1 tbsp
- Five-spice powder (optional), 1 tsp
- Teabags or maybe cheesecloth

Pho Aroma Combo:

- Ginger 2
- Star anise 4
- Cinnamon sticks 2
- Green cardamom 8
- Shallots 3 medium size
- Cilantro roots 4-5

Garnish:

- Lime wedges
- Bean sprouts
- Baby bok choy
- Red or green Fresno chili peppers
- Cilantro (optional)
- Mint leaves
- Hot chili pepper sauce (optional)
- Asian/Thai basil (optional)

Directions

Pre-Cooking:

1. Soak the dried shiitake mushrooms in room temperature water overnight. If you hurry on time, dip in warm temperature water till the mushrooms are smooth and tender.

2. Pre-boil the bones and the brisket: add the bones and the brisket to the broad pot and cover with water. Bring the water to a boil over high heat, reduce to low and simmer for another 10 minutes. Rinse the bones and beef over the room temperature of the tap water. Discard the broth.

3. Grill the ingredients in "Pho Aroma Combo" cast iron over medium flame. No oil has been applied. Rotate and flip the ingredients regularly so you can detect a sweet and lovely scent. Be alert that you do not burn the scent combo. The slightly burnt exterior surface is all right, just not fried.

4. Cut the mushrooms. Save the water from the mushroom. Approximately dice leek. Add the

scent combination and leeks to broad tea bags or cheesecloth bound with a cord.

Instant Pot Cooking:

1. In an instant pot of a 6-quarter scale, incorporate beef bones, brisket (fatty side up), sliced shiitake, diced carrots, scent combo, onion, and leeks (in tea bags). Stretch the mushroom water while you transfer the liquid to the pot. Flush the pot with more tap water before the 4-liter mark is hit. Seal the lid-Press Soup-Adjust to 40 minutes/High Pressure/More.

2. Enable the instant pot to release the natural pressure (the valve dropped), discard the entire onion and the scent combination in the tea bags.

3. Remove the brisket and soak it in cool water for at least 10 minutes. This would keep the meat from going black. Discard the fragrance and leek tea bags, the yellow onion, and the beef bones. Season the broth with 2 1/2 tsp of fine sea salt, 1 tsp of fish sauce and 1 tsp of five-spice powder (optional).

4. Slice the brisket at an angle of 45 degrees and toward the grain. Ladle the broth with bean sprouts, onions, mushrooms, mint leaves, Asian basil, chili peppers and sliced brisket. Serve heavy with the wedges of lime.

7.15-Minute Gazpacho along with Cucumber, Red Pepper and Basil

Servings: 4 | Prep Time: 15 Mins | Tot Time: 15 Mins

Ingredients

- Tomatoes, diced, 2¼ pounds
- Red bell pepper, diced, 1
- European cucumber, peeled and sliced, 1
- Garlic 1 clove
- Red onion, minced and divided, 1
- Chopped basil, divided, 4 tablespoons
- Kosher salt
- Ground black pepper
- Chopped cherry tomatoes 2 cups
- Olive oil 2 tablespoons

Directions

1. In a blender or a food processor dish, add peppers, red bell pepper, garlic, cucumber, half of the red onion and half of the basil. Puree the mixture until it is smooth.

2. Season the gazpacho with salt and pepper and mix.

3. Place the gazpacho in the bowls and marinade with the leftover onion and basil, the cherry tomatoes, and a slight drizzle of olive oil. Serve straight away.

8. Gluten-Free Mushroom Soup

Yield: 5 servings | Prep Time: 30 Mins | Total Time: 30 Mins

Ingredients

- Olive oil 1 tbsp
- Onion (diced) 1/2 large
- Mushrooms (sliced) 20 oz
- Garlic (minced) 6 cloves
- Chicken broth 2 cup

- Heavy cream 1 cup
- Almond milk (or coconut milk) 1 cup
- Sea salt 3/4 tsp
- Black pepper 1/4 tsp

Directions

1. In a wide pot over medium heat, sauté the onions and mushrooms in olive oil for around 10-15 minutes, stirring periodically, till lightly browned. Add the garlic and sauté for another minute.

2. Add chicken broth, cream, salt, almond milk, and black pepper. Carry to a boil, simmer for 15 minutes, stirring regularly.

3. Using a purée immersion blender until smooth (or puree in batches in a regular blender).

9. Instant-Pot Buffalo Chicken Soup

Servings: 2 | Prep Time: 10 Mins | Tot Time: 10 Mins

Ingredients

- Boneless and skinless chicken breasts 2

- Chicken bone broth 3 cups
- Diced Celery ½ cup
- Onion ¼ cup
- Garlic 1 clove
- Ranch dressing 1 tablespoon
- Butter 2 tablespoons
- Hot sauce 1/3 cup
- Cheddar cheese 2 cups
- Heavy cream 1 cup

Directions

1. Combine all ingredients EXCEPT cream & cheese in your pressure cooker.
2. Cook under pressure for ten min, then depressurize fast.
3. Carefully cut the chicken, shred, and go back to the broth. Remove heavy cream and cheese and mix to blend.

10. Creamy Avocado Cucumber Gazpacho

Servings: 6 | Prep Time: 15 Mins | Tot Time: 15 Mins

Ingredients

- Cucumbers 2 medium size
- Chopped avocado 1 ½
- Jalapeno 1 chopped
- Cilantro 1/3 cup
- Apple cider vinegar ¼ cup
- Garlic 2 cloves
- Salt 1 teaspoon
- Pepper ¾ teaspoon

- Water 1 to 1 ½ cups

Directions

1. In a blender or food processor, mix cucumber, avocado, cucumbers, cilantro, garlic, salt, vinegar, and pepper. Mix, so it's smooth.

2. Add 1 cup of water and mix, then add extra water to dilute if needed. Season with salt and pepper to taste.

11. Vegan Cauliflower Soup

Yield: 4-6 servings | Prep Time: 10 Mins | Total Time: 35 Mins

Ingredients

- Vegan butter ¼ cup
- Onion 1 large diced
- Garlic 3 cloves
- Cauliflower 1 large head
- Fresh thyme 1 teaspoon
- Water 5 cups
- Salt and pepper

- Lemon juice 1 small
- Vegan cream 1 cup

Directions

1. Prep: Begin by making the onion and garlic. Split the cauliflower into the bulbs, and they may be on the big side as you could split it down as it cooks.

2. Sauté: In a heavy bottom skillet, heat oil or water over medium heat, sauté the onion, after 6 minutes, add the garlic and cook for another 1 minute.

3. Add the remaining ingredients: cauliflower, thyme, a touch of salt and pepper and water/broth.

4. Simmer: carry the chunky soup to a boil, cover, minimize heat and simmer, stirring regularly, until the cauliflower is soft, about 20 minutes.

5. Add cream + lemon: stir in vegetable cream or vegetable milk and lemon juice.

6. Puree: After the soup is done, let it cool for 10 minutes. Puree the soup until optimal strength

using an immersion blender or cup blender. Dress with more salt and pepper as desired. Heat down before it warms up as desired.

7. Serve with a few allocated toasted cauliflower bits, a vegan cream drizzle, and/or new cracked pepper. Stir a little bit of red pepper flakes or crushed mustard seeds for a little spice. Mix with homemade Artisan Bread or fluffy and chewy Vegan Naan for juice soaking.

8. Store: The leftovers can be kept in the refrigerator for up to 6 days in a jar. For longer storage, freeze for up to 2 – 3 months.

12. Chicken Zucchini Noodle

Yield: 2-4 servings | Prep Time: 15 Mins | Total Time: 1 hour

Ingredients

- Diced red onion ½ heaping cup
- Celery ribs, diced, 2
- Carrot, diced, 1 large
- Garlic 2 cloves, minced

- Pinch of red pepper 1 small
- Fresh thyme 3 teaspoons
- Fresh oregano 3 teaspoons
- Chicken thighs, 4
- Bay leaves 2
- Chicken broth, 6 cups, low sodium
- Water 2 cups
- Zucchinis 3 medium

Directions

1. Put a big soup pot over medium heat and add the celery, onions, carrots, garlic, and red pepper flakes. Cook for 3-5 minutes or until vegetables and onions are translucent. Add thyme and oregano and simmer for another 1 minute, stirring constantly.

2. Put in the bay leaf and chicken thighs and pour in water, chicken broth, cover it, and bring it to a simmer. Boils reduce to a slow simmer and cook for 30 minutes. Within 30 minutes, cut the chicken and strip off the skin and dispose of it. Then shredded the chicken off the bone and put it aside with some juices. Put

the bones back in the soup pot and boil for another 10 minutes, uncovered.

3. Slice the zucchinis halfway lengthwise as the bones boil. And spiral them, using the Blade C. Set it aside.

4. Remove the bones and the bay leaves and dispose of them. Add the reserved shredded chicken and the zucchini noodles back to the cooker. Cook until the zucchini is al dente about 5 minutes or cooked according to your choice.

13. Instant Pot Butternut Squash

Servings: 4 | Prep Time: 10 Mins | Tot Time: 30 Mins

Ingredients

- Refined coconut oil 1½ tablespoons
- Yellow onion, diced, 1 large
- Red curry pastes ¼ cup
- Fresh ginger, grated, one 2-inch piece
- Garlic cloves, minced, 4 cloves
- Vegetable broth or water, 4 cups, low sodium

- Butternut squash, 1 medium, peeled
- Full-fat coconut milk one 13.5-ounce can
- Almond butter ¼ cup
- Reduced-sodium tamari 1 tablespoon
- Maple syrup or agave nectar 1 tablespoon
- Kosher salt, plus more to taste, 1 teaspoon
- Squeezed lime juice 3 teaspoons
- Fresh cilantro, sliced, plus more for garnishing, ½ cup
- Coconut yogurt, roasted peanuts, scallions, and sesame seeds, for serving

Directions

1. Pick the Sauté setting on the Instant Pot and add the coconut oil after a few minutes. When the oil is heavy, add the onion with a pinch of salt and cook until brown, for 6 to 7 minutes. Add curry paste, ginger, and garlic; simmer until very fragrant, constantly stirring for around 1 minute.
2. Spill in the broth and use a wooden spoon to scrape some browned pieces on the cup's

bottom. Add the coconut milk, butternut squash, tamarind, maple syrup, cashew butter, and salt. Stir to blend properly.

3. Secure the lid and add pressure to the Sealing. Pick the High-Pressure Soup setting and set the cooking time to 12 minutes.

4. When the timer is off, make a natural relaxation of the pressure for 5 minutes and rapidly release it.

5. Open the container and stir in the juice of the lime. Using an immersion blender, mix until the soup is smooth and fluffy. Alternatively, pass the soup to the blender using a dish towel to cover the blender cap to avoid steam from spreading.

6. When the broth has been purified, stir in the minced cilantro. Garnish with coconut yogurt, scallions, peanuts, and sesame seeds if needed.

14. Slow-Cooker Chicken Fajita Chili

Servings: 8 | Prep Time: 10 Mins | Tot Time: 6 hours

Ingredients

- Red bell pepper, diced, 1
- Green bell pepper, diced, 1
- Yellow bell pepper, diced, 1
- Onion, diced, 1
- Low-sodium black beans, 1 can
- Low-sodium pinto beans, 1 can, drained and rinsed
- Frozen yellow corn 1 package
- Low-sodium crushed tomatoes 1 can
- Low-sodium chicken broth 2 cups
- Chopped green chilies 1 can
- Cumin 2 tablespoons
- Chili powder 2 tablespoons
- Dried oregano 2 teaspoons
- Onion powder 1 tablespoon
- Garlic powder 1 tablespoon
- Red chili flakes ¼ teaspoon
- Boneless, skinless chicken breasts (about 3), 1½ pounds

- Juice of 1 lime (about 2 tablespoons)
- Fresh chopped cilantro 2 tablespoons

Directions

1. Mix all ingredients except lime juice and cilantro in a slow cooker and put the chicken on top. Cook on low for 6-8 hours or on high for 4-6 hours.
2. In the last 30 minutes of preparation, cut the chicken and sauté it. Return to a slow boiler with lime juice and cilantro and stir to combine.
3. Cook for another 30 minutes.
4. Serve with optional toppings as needed.

15. Cauliflower Soup along with Coconut, Turmeric and Lime

Servings: 4 | Prep Time: 10 Mins | Tot Time: 40 Mins

Ingredients

- Butter or ghee 2 tablespoons
- 2 sliced Leeks (white and light green part only)
- Finely chopped cilantro 1/3 cup
- Cauliflower, 1 1/2 pounds
- Ground turmeric 1/2 teaspoon
- Curry powder 2 tablespoons
- Sea salt
- Coconut milk, total 4 cups, 1 can
- Juice of 1 large lime

- Chopped cilantro

Directions

1. Melt the butter or ghee in a casserole over medium-low heat.
2. Add the leeks, cilantro, cauliflower, and sauté for 5 minutes.
3. Add turmeric, curry powder, and 1 1/2 teaspoon salt.
4. Pour in the coconut milk and stock, fire up to high and bring to a simmer.
5. Reduce heat to simmer, cover the pot partially and steam for 20-25 minutes until the cauliflower is tender.
6. Take a few cups of soup from the pot and stick it in a food processor or blender. Blend till smooth, then return to the jar.
7. Gently reheat and add the lime juice. Taste the salt and change it appropriately.
8. Top each bowl with the extra cilantro. Enjoy it.

Seafood and Fish

1. Dill Sauce with Trout or Salmon

Servings: 4 | Prep Time: 10 Mins | Tot Time: 15 Mins

Ingredients

Dill Sauce

- Lemon juice 1 - 2 tbsp.
- Lemon zest 1 tsp.
- Garlic powder 1/2 tsp.
- White sugar 1/2 tsp.
- Salt 1/4 - 1/2 tsp.
- Fresh dill (finely chopped), 2 1/2 tbsp.
- Milk 2 tbsp.
- Dijon (or hot English mustard) 2 tsp.
- Sour cream 3/4 cup

Fish

- Salt and pepper
- 4 salmon or the trout fillets (125g / 4oz each))
- 1/2 - 1 tbsp. of oil

Directions

1. Mix the elements of Dill Sauce (Mix well to loosen the sour cream). Adjust milk consistency and lemon juice tartness. Set at rest for 10 minutes - set aside for about 20 minutes if you're using fresh garlic.

2. Dry Pat Fish with a paper towel. Use salt and pepper to sprinkle.

3. In a skillet Heat the oil over medium-high heat. Place the fish side down in the skillet skin. Bake for about 2 minutes and then flip, then cook for 1 1/2 minutes on the other side.

4. Remove the serving plates from the skillet. End up serving with Dill Sauce, garnished with fresh dill and the lemon wedges if needed.

2. Salmon with a Bacon Tomato Sauce

Servings: 2 | Prep Time: 10 Mins | Tot Time: 25 Mins

Ingredients

Fish people Seafood Salmon

- 2-6 oz. filets Sockeye

Bacon Tomato with Vodka Cream Sauce

- Sliced garlic 1 clove
- 1 oz. Sliced onion
- Tomato paste (or simply 15 g) 1 tbsp.
- Olive oil 1 tsp.
- Lemon zest (grated) 1/2 tsp.
- Heavy cream (2-1/2 oz/75 ml) 1/3 cup
- Vodka (2 oz/ 60 ml) 1/4 cup
- Basil (chiffonade) 10 leaves
- Bacon (diced) 2 slices
- Water (1 oz/ 30 ml) 2 tbsp.
- Salt and pepper

Directions

1. Preparation: Allow the salmon to cool for 15 minutes on the counter. Collect all the ingredients. Now, slice the bacon.

2. Bacon: Over medium heat, put a frying pan (medium-sized). Add the 1 tsp of bacon oil and 1 tsp of oil and stir, covering the bacon.

Let them cook for 2 minutes. Meanwhile, dice the garlic and onion, slice the basil with the chiffonade and grate the lemon zest. (Stack the basil leaves for chiffonade, roll them longitudinally and then sliced crosswise, cut into thin ribbons.) Stir the bacon in the pan and cook unless browned and crisp. Cut the bacon so that the fat is left in a pan.

3. Salmon: But for about 2 tbsp., pour all the bacon fat out of the frying pan and return the pan over medium heat to the stove. Salt each salmon fillet relatively lightly and put them in a pan. Depending on the thickness, let it cook undisturbed for around 3-4 minutes. You're going to note the salmon get lighter, and it's going to let you judge whether it's time to flip. (Before tossing, you'll want the color to change about halfway.) Flip the fish with the spatula, then cook again for around 3-4 minutes. Remove the salmon gently with the foil to a plate and tent to stay warm.

4. Sauce: To keep the heat adjusted to just below medium, return the pan to the burner. Add the garlic and onions and mix until they

start to soften - around 1 1/2 minutes. Lift the pan from the burner, then pour the vodka slowly while standing back. Return the pan to heat, stirring to lift the browned pieces from the bottom of the pan. Let the vodka shrink in half.

5. To cook it up, cut it down, add the tomato paste and mix it around the onions. Add the water and heavy cream, swirling to mix. For a minute, let it simmer gently to thicken up a bit. Now add bacon, 1 tbsp of vodka, and lemon zest. Stir in the sauce until the alcohol's sharp scent has dissipated. Put some basil. Taste, and to the taste, add a pinch of salt and pepper. Switch the heat off.

6. Plate: On a serving plate, put a salmon fillet and top with the sauce. If needed, garnish it with more basil.

3. Skillet Salmon with an Avocado and Basil

Yield: 4 servings | Prep Time: 7 Mins | Total Time: 15 Mins

Ingredients

- ¼ cup basil (chopped)
- ¼ tsp. Ground black pepper
- ½ tsp. crushed red pepper
- 1 ½ tsp. coarse kosher salt (divided)
- 1 ½ lb. of boneless salmon filet (skin removed)
- 1 tbsp. lime juice
- 1 tsp. Italian seasonings
- 1 avocado
- 2 tsp. coconut oil
- chopped scallions (for garnish)

Directions

1. Heat oil over medium-high large skillet cast-iron skillet. Sprinkle all over the salmon with 3/4 tsp salt, crushed red pepper, Italian seasonings, and black pepper.

2. Lay salmon fillet skinned in the hot oil. Let cook until browned or crispy, and the meat is opaque or 4 to 6 minutes or depending on the thickness, around halfway up the side of the fillet. Flip over the salmon and remove the skillet from the heat.

3. Put the salmon in a hot pan, around 4 minutes more.

4. In the meantime, with basil and lime juice and the remaining 3/4 tsp salt, peel the pit and mash the avocado.

5. Serve salmon with avocado mash or sprinkled with the scallions When needed.

4. Keto Salmon Cakes

Yield: 2 servings | Prep Time: 4-5 Mins | Total Time: 6 Mins

Ingredients

Salmon cakes

- 1 tbsp. of avocado oil
- 1 egg
- 1/2 jalapeno, finely chopped
- 1/4 cup ground pork rinds
- 1/4 tsp. chili powder
- 1/4 tsp. garlic powder
- 2 tbsp. red onion (finely diced)
- 2 tbsp. of sarayo (or plain mayo)
- Salt and pepper
- Two 5 oz pouch of pink salmon (well-drained)

Avocado cream sauce

- 1/4 cup of sour cream
- 1-2 tbsp. of avocado oil
- 1-2 tsp. Water (to desired thickness)

- 1 avocado
- 3 tbsp. of cilantro
- Juice of a half lemon
- Salt & pepper to taste

Directions

1. Mix the salmon, egg, jalapeno, red onion, Sarayo, ground pork rinds and the seasoning in a big dish.
2. With combination, shape patties (4 large or 5-6 small)
3. Drizzle oil and fry patties over medium heat in a non-stick skillet for 4-5 minutes, until each side is lightly browned and crispy.

Avocado sauce

1. Blend all the food processor ingredients until fluffy.
2. Serve hot salmon cakes with the avocado sauce and sarayo with extra drizzle.

5. Two Salmon Tartare

Servings: 4 | Prep Time: 15 Mins | Tot Time: 2 hours 15 mins

Ingredients

- 450 g 1lb of fresh skinless salmon fillet
- 2 tbsp. of fresh lime juice
- 2 tbsp. of chopped green olives
- 2 tbsp. of capers chopped
- 150 g 5oz of smoked salmon
- 1/4 tsp. of freshly cracked black pepper
- 1/4 tsp. of **cayenne pepper**
- 1/4 cup of **paleo mayo**
- 1/4 cup of fresh parsley chopped
- 1/4 cup of **olive oil (extra-virgin)**
- 1 tsp. of **Dijon mustard**
- 1 tbsp. of caper brine

Directions

1. Cut a fresh salmon and a smoked salmon into very tiny 1/4-inch cubes using a sharp knife. Throw that along with the remaining

ingredients in a mixing bowl and mix finely until thoroughly mixed. Cover with the plastic film and put for about 2 hours in a refrigerator to marinate to make the solution to firm and completely meld the flavors.

2. Divide the salmon into 4 equal servings until ready to eat and force each serving into a circular cookie cutter. Lightly pack the fish with a spoon and cut the seal.

3. If needed, garnish with the fresh herbs and a drizzle of olive oil (extra-virgin).

4. Serve with something crunchy such as crackers, Tostones, or fresh veggies.

6. Baked Salmon & Asparagus in Foil

Servings: 4 | Prep Time: 10 Mins | Tot Time: 30 Mins

Ingredients

- 1 lb. asparagus (trim the tough ends)
- 1 lemon (thinly sliced)
- 2-1/2 Tbsp. of olive oil
- 4 (6 oz) salmon fillets (skinless)

- 2 cloves of minced garlic
- Fresh dill sprigs (can use chopped fresh rosemary, thyme, or parsley)
- Salt & ground black pepper

Directions

1. Preheat the oven to 400°F. Cut the four sheets of

    approximately 14-inch-long aluminum foil. Divide the asparagus into four equal portions (approximately 8 spears per packet of foil) and the center layer of each foil length.

2. Mix the oil with the garlic in a small bowl. Drizzle the asparagus portion with 1 tsp of oil, then sprinkle with the salt & pepper. Rinse the salmon, remove the excess water, and add salt & pepper to the bottom of every fillet.

3. Drizzle 1 tsp of an olive oil mixture on top of each salmon fillet and season with salt & pepper to taste. Top each with around 2 dill sprigs and 2 lemon slices

4. Wrap the foil sides inward around the salmon and fold the foil top and bottom to enclose.

5. On a baking sheet, put foil pouches in a single layer. Cook in a preheated oven unless the salmon is fully cooked, about 25 to 30 minutes. Finally, Unwrap, then serve warm.

7. Keto Salmon & Gluten Free Tzatziki Cucumber Noodles

Servings: 2 | Prep Time: 10 Mins | Tot Time; 30 Mins

Ingredients

For the tzatziki sauce:

- kosher salt (to taste)
- 140 g Greek-style yogurt
- 1-2 cloves garlic grated
- 1 tsp. fresh dill (or only 3/4 tsp. dried)
- 1 tbsp. white wine vinegar
- 1 tbsp. lemon juice
- 1 tbsp. extra virgin olive oil
- 1 cucumber spiralized (or grated)

For the salmon:

- 1 tbsp. extra virgin olive oil
- 1 tsp. freshly grated lemon zest
- 2 cloves garlic grated
- 2 salmon fillets about 5 oz. each (With skins)
- freshly ground pepper (to taste)
- kosher to taste

Directions

For the tzatziki sauce:

1. Mix the yogurt, olive oil, lemon juice, garlic, vinegar, and dill in a medium bowl, then season to taste. If the cucumber is grating, add it in and leave it out if it is spiralizing. Refrigerate until needed while covered.

For the salmon:

1. Preheat the oven to 400 ºF/200 ºC.
2. In a pan, mix the olive oil, lemon zest, garlic, and season to taste.
3. A large piece of foil is very lightly oiled (about twice the salmon filets' size). Place the salmon skin's side over the foil and brush with the

olive oil on the garlic. To create an envelope, fold the foil to (or in whatever shape you desire, if it is sealed closed).

4. Place the foil packet on the rimmed baking sheet and bake for 16-20 minutes until cooked

5. **OPTIONAL**: change the oven settings to broil and cook the salmon for 3-4 minutes to crisp up the top (tin foil open).

6. Using a spatula, remove the salmon from the foil. The skins will stand to the foil, and in one piece, the fillets will come out.

7. Serve over a bed of cucumber noodles right away and top off with the tzatziki sauce.

8. Superb Salmon Ceviche

Servings: 4 | Prep Time: 5 Mins | Tot Time: 35 Mins

Ingredients

- Salt and pepper
- Large lettuce leaves to serve in
- Juice of 1 lime
- A handful of sesame seeds (toasted)

- A handful of coriander leaves
- 400 g of salmon fillet skinned
- 2 spring onions (diagonally chopped)
- 1/4 cucumber of finely cubed
- 1 tsp. Of sesame oil
- 1 tsp. Of rapeseed oil
- 1 tsp. Ginger (finely grated)

Directions

1. The salmon must be half-frozen because it's easier to carve. Usefully frozen fillets of salmon, which aren't too thick, or it is tough to cover them. Ideally, before cutting, stick them for half an hour in the fridge (0.5 cm square should be the cubes).

2. Grate the ginger with it.

3. In a bowl place the salmon pieces and add the grated ginger to the lime juice. Ensure that it is adequately coated. Until eating, chill for about 1/2 hour so that the salmon will "cook" in lime juice.

4. Roast the sesame seeds in a skillet (low heat), move them around periodically so that they are brown, but don't burn

5. Cube the cucumber and dice the spring onions. Add the cucumber, tomatoes, coriander, and oil after the salmon is refrigerated for 1/2-hour, season with salt & pepper, and mix gently.

9. Roasted Salmon with a Parmesan Dill Crust

Yield: 2 servings | Prep Time: 2 Mins | Total Time: 12 Mins

Ingredients

- ¼ cup parmesan cheese (grated)
- ¼ cup of mayonnaise
- 1 tbsp. dill weed
- 1 tsp. ground mustard
- 2 pieces of salmon about 1.5lbs

Directions

1. Preheat the oven to 450°F.

2. Mix the mayonnaise, the parmesan cheese, the dill, and the mustard.

3. Take a foil-lined baking sheet and place the salmon on it.

4. On top of each slice of salmon, smear half of a mayonnaise mixture.

5. For around 10 minutes, roast in the oven until the crust becomes brown and the fishes flakes instantly.

10. Walnut (Maple) Crusted Salmon

Servings: 4 | Prep Time: 10 Mins | Tot Time: 3 hours

Ingredients

- Sprinkle of **salt** & pepper
- 4 - 6oz salmon fillets
- 2 tbsp. of **ghee**

Walnut Crust

- 3 tbsp. **pure maple syrup**
- 1/2 tsp. **onion powder**
- 1/2 tsp. **cracked black pepper**
- 1/2 tsp. of **chipotle powder**
- 1/2 cup **walnuts** (finely chopped)
- 1 tsp. **smoked paprika**
- 1 tsp. **coconut aminos**
- 1 tbsp. of **apple cider vinegar**

Directions

1. To a small bowl, add the ingredients and stir when well mixed.
2. Put the salmon fillets and spoon a mixture over each fish piece on a pan, spreading it as equally as you can. Place, uncovered, in the refrigerator for 2 - 3 hours.

3. Preheat the oven to 425 ºF.

4. In a large oven-safe skillet set at high heat, melt the ghee. Add the fish pieces, then let them cook uninterrupted for around 2 minutes when the pan is warm so that the skin is fair.

5. Move the pan to the oven and, depending on the preferred thickness and the thickness of these fillets, keep cooking these fish for around 5-8 minutes.

6. Drizzle before serving, if desired, with a little melted ghee and extra maple syrup.

11. Sweet Chili Salmon

Yield: 4 servings | Prep Time: 2 Mins | Total Time: 12 Mins

Ingredients

- 1/2 cup of sweet chili sauce
- 1/4 cup of lime juice
- 2 tbsp. of olive oil
- 4 salmon fillets (150 grams/6 oz.)

Directions

1. In a small cup blend together the olive oil and lime juice.

2. Add the salmon in the paste and coat both ends.

3. Oiled the large frying pan with olive oil and heat to medium. Add the salmon, keep the skin side down, to the hot pan until hot. Until tossing and frying for another 5 minutes, sear for 5 minutes.

4. Take from an oven and let sit before drizzling with the sweet chili sauce for 1 minute.

12. Salmon Meatballs with Garlic Lemon Cream Sauce

Yield: 20 servings | Prep Time: 10-15 Mins | Total Time: 35-40 Mins

Ingredients

- 2 tbsp. **Organic Grass-Fed Butter (or ghee** or ghee/coconut oil)
- 2 cloves **Garlic**
- 1 lb. **ground wild salmon**

- 2 tbsp. **Dijon mustard**
- 1 large egg
- 1 tbsp. **organic coconut flour**
- 1 tsp. **homemade seasoned salt**
- 1/3 cup **Onion**
- 1/4 cup chopped fresh Chives

For the Lemon Cream Sauce

- 1 medium **lemon(s)** Juiced & zested
- 2 cups **Heavy Cream, A2 Pasture Raised** or coconut cream
- 2 tbsp. **Dijon mustard**
- 2 tbsp. **Organic Grass-Fed Butter or Ghee** or ghee/coconut oil
- 2+ tbsp. Fresh Chives, chopped
- 4 cloves **Garlic**

Directions

1. Preheat the oven to 350 ºF.
2. Sauté the onions and garlic in the butter until tender, around 3 minutes, over medium heat in a deep skillet. Enable to cool and put aside.

3. Mix the remaining meatball ingredients with the fried onion mixture in a large bowl and mix properly.

4. Bake For 20-25 minutes at 350 or until as required.

5. Create the cream sauce while the meatballs are frying.

6. Sauté the garlic in the butter until tender, around 3 minutes, in a large skillet over medium heat.

7. Put the Dijon mustard and lemon juice and whisk until mixed. A hard cream whisk. Simmer until you reach the desired thickness, stirring regularly.

8. Taking the fried meatballs out of the oven, then put them in the sauce. Decorate with chives.

9. Serve the cream sauce meatballs and enjoy

13. Baked Cod

Yield: 2 servings | Prep Time: 15 Mins | Total Time: 40 Mins

Ingredients

- 12 oz. cod, cut into 4 equal fillets
- 1/3 cup finely grated parmesan cheese
- 1 tbsp. chopped fresh parsley
- 1/2 tsp. smoked paprika
- 1/4 tsp. table salt
- For the Sauce:
- 4 cloves garlic (minced)
- 1/4 cup dry white wine
- 2 tbsp. fresh lemon juice
- 1 tbsp. salted butter

Directions

1. Prepare: preheat to 400 ºF and put an oven rack in the oven's center. Using the paper towels, dry Pat Cod fillets. Sprinkle each fillet's both sides with salt. And put aside.

2. For the sauce: Melt the butter in an oven-proof pan over medium heat, then stirring continuously for less than a minute. Stir in the minced garlic for 1 to 2 minutes before it is aromatic and begins to brown. To the bowl,

add some white wine and lemon juice. They need to start to boil immediately. Stir briefly, then switching the heat off.

3. Add Cod: Whisk the parmesan cheese with the paprika in a mixing bowl until well-mixed. Place the cod fillets side by side over the sauce in the skillet. Spoon the parmesan blend generously over the top of the fillets in the skillet, using a spoon to fan it out until uniformly spread over the fillets. If the parmesan comes off the fillets, it's okay because it will become part of the sauce.

4. Bake: Move the pan to the oven until the oven has heated until 400 degrees F. Cook for 15 to 20 minutes until the cod fillets become cooked.

5. Serve: Use a spatula to gently move the cod fillets to serve dishes, to prevent upsetting the topping of parmesan. Stir together the remaining liquid in a pan, cook for a minute over medium-high heat to thicken the sauce, and drizzle the sauce over the fish. Sprinkle on top of parsley and serve while it is hot.

14. Parmesan Baked Cod

Servings: 4 | Prep Time: 10 Mins | Tot Time: 25 Mins

Ingredients

- lemon wedges (cut into wedges)
- 4 cod fillets - about 6 oz. each
- 2 tsp. paprika
- 1 tbsp. extra virgin olive oil
- 1 tbsp. chopped parsley (or 1 tsp. dried parsley)
- ¾ cup fresh Parmesan cheese (grated)
- ¼ tsp. sea salt

Directions

1. Preheat the oven to 400 ºF. Top with parchment paper or foil on a baking sheet.
2. Blend the parmesan, parsley, paprika, and salt in a small dish. Drizzle some cod with olive oil, then dredge the mixture with the cheese and gently press it with the fingertips. Move to the tray for baking. Cover the cod with some combination of leftover cheese.

3. Bake in the thickest portion until the fish becomes opaque, 10-15 minutes. Then serve with slices of lemon.

15. Buttered Cod in Skillet

Servings: 4 | Prep Time: 5 Mins | Tot Time: 10 Mins

Ingredients

cod-

- 6 Tbsp. unsalted butter (sliced)
- 1 1/2 lbs. cod fillets

seasoning-

- Parsley, herbs, or cilantro
- few lemons slice
- ¾ tsp. of **ground paprika**
- ½ tsp. **salt**
- ¼ tsp. of ground black pepper
- ¼ tsp. of **garlic powder**

Directions

1. In a deep bowl, stir the seasoning ingredients together.

2. When desired, cut the cod into smaller bits. Season the seasoning with all the sides of the cod.

3. Heat 2 Tbsp of butter on medium-high heat in the large skillet. Add the cod to the skillet until the butter melts. 2 minutes to cook.

4. Switch down the heat to mild. Switch the cod over, add the butter's remainder and cook for a further 3-4 minutes.

5. The butter will melt entirely, and a fish will be fried. (Do not overcook the cod, it is indeed going to get mushy and fall apart entirely.)

6. Drizzle the fresh lemon juice with the fish. Floor, if needed, with fresh herbs. Immediately serve.

16. Simple Garlic Shrimp Alfredo with Zoodles

Servings: 2 | Prep Time 10 Mins | Tot Time: 20 Mins

Ingredients

- 4 cooked bacon strips (chopped)
- 3 mediums julienned, zucchini or spiralized

- 2 Tbsp. garlic
- 1/4 cup of parmesan cheese
- 1/4 cup butter
- 1/3 cup heavy cream
- 1/2 tsp. sea salt
- 1/2 tsp. of fresh cracked pepper
- 1 tsp. paprika
- 1 lbs. shrimp (peeled and deveined)

Directions

1. Melt the butter in a decent cookie skillet over medium-high heat.
2. Toss in the garlic and shrimp while bubbling. Sprinkle with flour, paprika and pepper. When cooked through, cook on both sides.
3. Move it with a slotted spoon to a dish. Place the zucchini in the pan and drizzle with the milk. Simply cook until hot. Retract from the heat.
4. Using parmesan to sprinkle. Serve with shrimp topping.

17. Keto & Paleo Pad Thai With the Shirataki Noodles

Yield: 2 servings | Prep Time: 5 Mins | Total Time: 30 Mins

Ingredients

- 2-3 tbsp. fresh lime juice
- 1/4 tsp. blackstrap molasses
- 1/8-1/4 tsp. cayenne pepper (or red pepper flakes)
- 1 1/2 tbsp. fish sauce
- 1 1/2 tbsp. coconut aminos
- 1-2 tbsp. coconut oil
- 1 package of shirataki fettuccini noodles
- 2 tbsp. xylitol or erythritol
- 2 cloves of garlic minced
- 200 g of fresh shrimp (you can also use chicken)
- 2 lightly beaten eggs
- 30 g of bean sprouts

For serving:

- ½ cup of cilantro leaves torn
- 3 finely sliced green onions
- 35 g unsalted peanuts (toasted & roughly chopped)
- lime wedges

Directions

Preparation of the shirataki noodles

1. Drain the noodles, rinse well with cold water, put them in the boiling water for about two minutes, and dry the noodles over medium heat in a non-oiled pan. Now put it aside.

Preparation of the keto pad Thai

2. In a small cup, thoroughly whisk together fish sauce, amino coconut, sweetener, red pepper flakes or cayenne. Starting at 2 tsp. Add lime juice to taste.
3. Heat oil in a skillet or pan (medium heat). Add garlic and sauté briefly before the browning begins. Add in the shrimp and cook on each side for 2-5 minutes. On the side of the dish, pile the shrimp.
4. Pour in the gently beaten eggs, cook until firm but still moist and soft, and stir them to scramble.
5. Pour in the cooked sauce and blend briefly until finely mixed with the shrimp and the scrambled eggs. Put in

the seasoned noodles and toss in the sauce to coat. Add the soy sprouts and keep cooking for 2-3 minutes.

6. Add green onions, peanuts, and cilantro to garnish. Serve with new lime promptly.

18. Lobster Tails with a Garlic Butter

Servings: 2 | Prep Time: 10 Mins | Tot Time: 15 Mins

Ingredients

- Juice of a **lemon**
- 5 cloves minced **garlic**
- 4 tbsp. of **melted butter**
- 2 (8oz) **lobster tails**
- 1/4 cup grated **Parmesan**

- 1 tsp. of **Italian seasoning**

Directions

1. Preheat the oven to 400°F. Mix the garlic, parmesan, Italian seasoning, lemon juice, and melted butter in a medium bowl and season with salt.

2. Cut the translucent skin off the lobster and rub the lobster tails with both garlic butter seasoning, using sharp scissors.

3. Place the lobster tails and bake these lobster tails for 12 to 15 minutes on a parchment-lined baking sheet. The lobster meat would be stable and opaque inside. The internal temperature should be between 140 °F - 145 °F.

19. Avocado Tuna Melt

Servings: 4 | Prep Time: 10 Mins | Tot Time: 20 Mins

Ingredients

- 1 can tuna
- 1 tsp. paprika

- 1/2 cup of cheddar cheese (shredded)
- 1/4 cup mayonnaise
- 1/4 cup of onion (finely diced)
- 1/4 cup of pickles (finely diced)
- 1/4 cup of red bell pepper (finely diced)
- 2 avocadoes
- salt & pepper to taste

Directions

1. Preheat the oven to 400°F/200°C.
2. To make the hole even smaller, scoop out some avocado. In the tuna salad, mix a bit of scooped avocado.
3. Mix the salmon, tomato, pickle, red bell pepper, cheese, paprika, and mayo. With the salt and pepper, season to the taste.
4. Scoop in the avocado with the tuna mixture and finish with more cheese.
5. keep for about 5-10 minutes in the oven until cheese melts.

20. Keto Tuna Casserole

Yield: 2 servings | Prep Time: 15 Mins | Total Time: 30 Mins

Ingredients

- ¼ cup of chopped parsley (for garnish0
- ¼ cup of minced red onion
- ¼ tsp. black pepper
- ¼ tsp. cayenne pepper
- ¼ tsp. sea salt
- ⅓ cup avocado oil mayonnaise
- ½ cup gruyere cheese (shredded, divided)
- 1 tbsp. Dijon mustard
- 2 (5 oz) cans of tuna in water (drained)

Directions

1. Preheat to 400ºF in the oven.
2. The salmon, mayonnaise, vinegar, 1/4 cup of cheese, tomato, pepper, cayenne, and salt are blended.

3. In a little casserole dish, put the mixture. Sprinkle on top of the remaining 1/4 cup of melted cheese.

4. Bake for around 15 minutes. Sprinkle with the parsley and eat promptly and scoop out with cut-up vegetables and pork rinds.

21. Gluten Free, Low Carbohydrate Keto Chips & Fish

Yield: 2 servings | Prep Time: 20 Mins | Total time: 2 hours

Ingredients

For the gluten-free & keto fish tacos

- 250 g firm white-flesh fish (preferably cod)
- 2 tsp. apple cider vinegar
- 4 cloves garlic (ran through a press)
- kosher salt to taste
- 1 tsp. baking powder
- 1 egg
- 1 tbsp. sour cream (or coconut cream)
- 2 tsp. apple cider vinegar

- coconut oil (or cooking oil of choice)
- 1/2 cup of whey protein isolate
- 1/4 - 1/2 tsp. kosher salt (to taste)
- 1/3 cup sour cream
- 1/4 tsp. garlic powder

Serving suggestions

- Vinegar
- Lemon
- 1 batch keto mayonnaise
- 1 batch jicama fries (8 tortillas)

Directions

1. Mix up the sour cream (or coconut) with the garlic, vinegar, and season with salt to taste. Cut the fish into slices about 2 inches wide across the flesh's grain and introduce them a cream marinade. NOW Cover and refrigerate, preferably overnight, for two hours.
2. Make the keto jicama fries in a batch.
3. To make it around half-inch deep, prepare the frying station by applying enough oil to the skillet or pan. Using a smaller pan and fry in

batches will save a lot of oil. up When coating the cod, heat the oil over medium-low heat.

4. In a small dish or platter, blend the whey protein, garlic powder, baking powder, and salt. Whisk the egg with the cream and vinegar on a second plate or a dish.

5. Coat the fish by gently scraping the excess marinade, then dip in the egg mixture, followed by the mixture of whey protein, putting immediately in the hot oil, then basting immediately on the top. For maximum crispness, you want to fry fish after coating it. Fry until deeply golden on both sides and move to a paper-lined sheet for a few minutes.

6. Serve over a jicama fries' bed, mayonnaise, plenty of lemons and a splash of vinegar right now.

22. Tuna Cakes

Servings: 4 | Prep Time: 10 Mins | Tot Time: 30 Mins

Ingredients

- 1 Egg
- 1 Garlic Clove (Minced)
- 1 Red Pepper (Finely Diced)
- 1 tsp. Paprika
- 1 Yellow Onion (Finely Diced)
- 1/2 Lime (Juice)
- 1/2 tbsp. Salt
- 1/2 tsp. Black Pepper
- 1/4 cup Chopped Fresh Chives
- 2 Sweet Potato (Around 2 Cups Chopped)

- 3 cans of tuna

Directions

1. Chop the sweet potato in small cubes and let it boil in salted water for 10 minutes. They ought to be fork tender.

2. Sauté the finely diced red pepper and onion in some oil while the potato boils, until the onion is tender.

3. Now, in a mixing bowl, mix all this until well mixed. To smash the potato, use a wooden spoon, which leaves it slightly chunky.

4. Make the mixture into cakes for fish. Using 1/4 of a cup per cake, which resulted in 12 cakes.

5. Heat oil over medium-high heat in a skillet. Place the fish cakes carefully in the pan, but once the pan is hot and lets them get a nice sear on each side. Leave them sit side by side for a minimum of 3 minutes. Chop the sweet potato in small cubes and let it boil in salted water for 10 minutes. They ought to be fork tender.

a. Sauté the finely diced red pepper and onion in some oil while the potato boils, until the onion is tender.

b. Now, in a mixing bowl, mix all this until well mixed. To smash the potato, use a wooden spoon, which leaves it slightly chunky.

c. Make the mixture into cakes for fish. Use 1/4 of a cup per cake, which resulted in 12 cakes.

d. Heat oil over medium-high heat in a skillet. Place the fish cakes carefully in the pan once the pan is hot and let them get a nice sear on each side. Let them sit side by side for a minimum of 3 minutes.

23. Keto Fish Pie

Servings: 6 | Prep Time: 15 Mins | Tot Time: 1 hour 15 mins

Ingredients

- 3 cloves
- 3 bay leaves
- 200g g salmon fillets (cubed and skinless)

- 200 g white fish (cubed and skinless)
- 2 cups cheddar cheese
- 100g g smoked whitefish (mackerel, haddock, or similar)
- 100 g butter
- 1/2 cup whole milk
- 1/2 cup peas
- 1 tsp. Dijon mustard
- 1 small bunch fresh parsley (around 20g)
- 1 pinch nutmeg
- 1 onion (chopped)
- 1 large cauliflower (2lb)
- 1 cup spinach
- 1 cup of heavy whipping cream

Directions

1. Preheat the oven up to 390 °F or 200 °C
2. Begin the topping with the Cauliflower. For 10 minutes, cut into small pieces and steam. Take from the steam and allow the water to evaporate from the Cauliflower for a few

minutes then you can put it in a food processor. Add a pinch of salt and 50g of butter and mix until smooth. Put it aside.

3. In a medium-heat pan, add the sauce while the Cauliflower becomes steaming. Put the butter, bay leaves and chopped onion in the mixture. Fry until the onion is opaque but not browned, for 5 minutes.

4. Move to a boil and add the milk, cream, and cloves. Return the fish and poach to the pan, frequently stirring, on low heat for about 10 minutes.

5. Using a slotted spoon to get the fish from the pan and move it into the baking dish in which you will bake the pie. The sauce begins to boil, moving it to a medium flame.

6. Drop from the sauce the cloves and bay leaves and include the 1 and 1/2 cups of cheddar, a pinch of nutmeg powder and Dijon mustard.

7. Add the spinach, parsley, and peas to the sauce after the cheese melted in the sauce and put it down to a boil for about 5 minutes, stirring frequently.

8. Get the pie packed now. Pour over the fish with the sauce and blend to mix. Cover with Cauliflower's mash, then drag a fork's prongs across the mash to roughen the surface. Sprinkle with the leftover cheddar cheese, then bake until the cheese becomes golden brown and bubbling on top for 25-30 minutes.

9. Let the pie cool for about 10-15 minutes and serve with a fresh parsley garnish. Serve instantly or leave to cool and remain in the refrigerator for up to 4 days.

24. Salmon in a Roasted Pepper Sauce

Yield: 2 servings | Prep Time: 5 Mins | Total Time: 25 Mins

Ingredients

- Salt & pepper to taste
- Salt & pepper to season
- 4 oz. of roasted red peppers (diced)
- 4 cups baby spinach
- 3 cloves garlic (finely diced)
- 2 salmon fillets with skin (about 1 lb.)

- 1/4 tsp. of red pepper flakes
- 1/4 cup of grated Parmesan cheese
- 1/4 cup parsley (chopped)
- 1/2 cup Half & Half (or heavy cream)
- 1 tbsp. olive oil
- 1 tbsp. butter

Directions

1. With salt and black pepper, season these salmon fillets.

2. Over a low boil, heat the oil in the medium-sized non-stick skillet. Cook the flesh-side down salmon fillets first, for about 5 minutes on either side or cooked at the preference. Remove these from the pan until cooked and put aside.

3. Add the butter and garlic to the same plate. Cook for about 1 minute, then include the roasted peppers and cook for an additional 2 minutes.

4. Add and encourage the spinach to wilt.

5. Mix Half Parmesan, parsley, red pepper flakes, salt, and pepper and turn the heat down to medium. Move to a boil and stir.

6. Put the salmon back in the pan and spoon over each fillet with the sauce.

7. Serve over vegetables such as spaghetti, potatoes, or steamed.

25. Keto Fried Fish

Servings: 4 | Prep Time: 15 Mins | Tot Time: 30 Mins

Ingredients

- Avocado oil
- 4 (6 oz) thin fillets (of a white fish such as cod or sole)
- 1/2 tsp. garlic powder

- 1/2 tsp. dried thyme
- 1/2 tsp. black pepper
- 1 tsp. kosher salt (diamond crystal)
- 1 large egg
- 1 cup blanched almond flour (finely ground)

Directions

1. Whisk the eggs with salt, garlic powder, pepper, and dried thyme in a small dish.

2. In the egg mixture, dip the fish fillet. Put it on the cutting board and sprinkle with the almond flour (1/4 cup per fillet) and press to make the coating adhere to both sides' fingertips. This process works better than dredging fish in almond flour since the almond flour left in the bowl gets soggy and oily and almost useless when dredging.

3. Pour avocado oil, hit around 1/2 inch thick, into a large non-stick frying pan. Heat until hot or for 3-5 minutes on medium-high heat.

4. Put the fillets in a pan carefully. (work in batches if necessary). Cook for 3-4 minutes, until the bottom, becomes crisp.

5. Flip with the fish. Lower-to-medium heat. Cook until cooked through and crisp, 3-4 more minutes.

Vegan and vegetarian recipes

1. Ratatouille

Yield: 4 servings | Prep Time: 30 Minutes | Total Time: 50 Minutes

Ingredients

- Pinch of red pepper flakes (crushed)
- Kosher salt
- Freshly ground black pepper
- Extra-virgin olive oil (divided)
- Crusty baguette
- Bunch of fresh basil
- 3 cloves garlic
- 2 zucchinis (sliced into 1/4 "coins)
- 2 media eggplant (diced into 1/2" pieces)
- 2 bell peppers (cut into ¼ inch spears
- 2 cup halved cherry tomatoes
- 1/2 cup dry white wine

- 1 large onion (chopped)
- 1 bay leaf
- 1 tsp. Dried oregano
- 1 tbsp. Tomato paste

Directions

1. In a colander, put the eggplant and toss it with a large pinch of salt. Leave the eggplant at rest for around 20 minutes, and pat it dry to remove excess moisture.

2. Heat 1 tbsp oil in the oven or a big kettle. Add the eggplant, then season with pepper and salt. Cook all over until golden (around 6 minutes) and remove the eggplant.

3. Apply the pot to the remaining tbsp of oil. Add the onion, bay leaf, and bell peppers, and cook for about 5 minutes, stirring regularly, before the onion and peppers become tender.

4. Add the tomato paste and whisk until the paste is fragrant for around 1 minute, now deglaze a pan with white wine until much of the liquid becomes evaporated. Stir in the zucchini and simmer for around 4 more

minutes, until tender. Stir in the garlic, oregano, and cherry tomatoes.

5. Season a mixture with salt & pepper and red pepper flakes and boil until the tomatoes begin to cut down, stirring periodically.

6. Back to the pot, add the eggplant and stir to mix. Garnish with the basil, and then serve warm with a baguette.

2. Whole Roasted Cauliflower

Servings: 4 | Prep Time: 15 Mins | Tot Time: 1 hour 15 mins

Ingredients

- 1/8 tsp. paprika
- 1 medium head cauliflower (around 2 1/4 lbs.)
- 1/4 cup fresh flat-leaf parsley (chopped)
- 1/4 tsp. red pepper flakes (crushed)
- 1/4 tsp. ground black pepper (Freshly)
- 1/2 tsp. kosher salt (divided)
- 2 pt. cherry (or grape tomatoes)

- 4 tbsp. extra-virgin olive oil (divided)
- 4 cloves garlic (smashed and peeled)

Directions

1. While keeping the rack in the center, preheat the oven to 400 °F. Place the tomatoes & garlic, drizzle with 3 tbsp of oil in a bread baking dish, and then sprinkle with a 1/4 tsp. Salt, red pepper, and pepper flakes. Toss it to coat it.

2. Trim and discard the cauliflower's broad green leaves, then trim the stem such that the cauliflower lies flat. Put it aside the tomatoes and put the cauliflower in the center of the platter. Drizzle the cauliflower with the remaining tbsp of oil and add to the coat. Sprinkle with the paprika and 1/4 tsp. of the remaining salt. Roast for around 1 hour, or before a paring knife makes the cauliflower soft and quick to pierce.

3. Sprinkle over the cauliflower with parsley. Cut the cauliflower into wedges, then serve with garlic and tomatoes.

3. Best Arugula Salad

Yield: 2 servings | Prep Time: 5 Mins | Total Time: 5 Mins

Ingredients

For Dressing

- 2 tbsp. lemon juice
- 4 cup arugula Shaved Parmesan (for garnish)
- 6 tbsp. extra-virgin olive oil
- Kosher salt & ground black pepper

Directions

1. Making of dressing: whisk together the olive oil and the lemon juice in a medium cup, and season with salt & pepper.
2. Dress the arugula gently in a wide bowl, then line it with parmesan.

4. Roasted Brussels Sprouts

Servings: 4 | Prep Time: 5 Mins | Tot Time: 30 Mins

Ingredients

- Kosher salt
- Ground black pepper
- Flaky sea salt (for serving)
- Olive oil 2 tbsp.
- Brussels sprouts (trimmed and halved) 1 lb.

Directions

1. Preheat the oven to 425 °F. Sprinkle the Brussels sprouts with olive oil on a big baking sheet and season with salt and pepper. Toss together when merged.

2. keep roasting until the Brussels sprouts on the outside are crispy and soft inside, shaking the pan partly for about 25 minutes.

3. Sprinkle, if necessary, with flaky sea salt and serve immediately.

5. Instant - Pot Vegetable Soup

Yield: 6 servings | Prep Time: 10 Mins | Total Time: 45 Mins

Ingredients

- Kosher salt
- ground black pepper
- chopped parsley (for serving)
- 4 garlic cloves (minced)
- 4 cup low-sodium vegetable broth
- 3/4 tsp. paprika
- 2 celery stalks (thinly sliced)
- 2 carrots (peeled and thinly sliced)
- 2 tsp. Italian seasoning
- 2 cup small cauliflower florets

- 2 cup chopped cabbage
- 1 red bell pepper (chopped)
- 1 medium zucchini (chopped)
- 1 medium onion (chopped)
- 1 (15-oz.) Can of kidney beans (rinsed and drained)
- 1 (15-oz.) can diced tomatoes
- 1 tbsp. tomato paste
- 1 tbsp. extra-virgin olive oil (plus more for serving)

Directions

1. Add the oil, garlic, and onion and set the Instant Pot to 'Sauté.' With salt & pepper, season generously. Cook until the onion softens, stirring regularly, for 5 minutes. Add the tomato paste and simmer for 1 minute, stirring. Add the rest ingredients and stir.
2. Lock the lid and load the machine to cook for 12 minutes under high pressure. Turn the steam valve carefully to a venting position when finished for releasing the pressure.
3. Dress with salt & pepper and stir in the soup.

4. Until serving, garnish it with parsley and the drizzle of olive oil.

6. Easiest-Ever Guacamole

Yield: 6 servings | Prep Time; 10 Mins | Total Time: 10 Mins

Ingredients

- 1 small, minced jalapeño (seeded if you prefer less heat)
- 1/2 tsp. kosher salt
- 1/2 small of white onion (finely chopped)
- 1/4 cup chopped cilantro (also for garnish)
- 3 avocados pitted
- Juice of 2 limes

Directions

1. Combine the avocados, lime juice, onion, jalapeño, salt, and cilantro, in a wide dish.
2. Stir, then turn the bowl gently as you run the fork over the avocados (it will ensure that the mixture remains chunky) until the desired consistency has been met. If necessary,

season with more salt. Before serving, garnish it with more cilantro.

7. Zucchini Cauliflower Fritters

Yield: 8 servings | Prep Time: 5 Mins | Total Time: 10 Mins

Ingredients

Original version

- 2 medium zucchinis
- 2 large eggs
- 1/4 tsp black pepper
- 1/4 cup of coconut flour
- 1/2 tsp sea salt
- 1/2 head chopped cauliflower (approximately 3 cups)

Egg-Free version

- 2 medium zucchinis
- 1/4 tsp black pepper
- 1/4 cup flour (all-purpose flour, gluten-free if needed)

- 1/2 tsp sea salt
- 1/2 head chopped cauliflower (approximately 3 cups)

Directions

1. In the food processor or a high-speed blender, grate the zucchini.
2. For about 5 minutes, steam the cauliflower until just fork tender. In the food processor/blender, add the cauliflower and process until it is broken down into tiny chunks. But don't over process because it will turn into a mash.
3. Squeeze that much moisture as feasible out of the grated vegetables using a dishtowel or almond milk bag.
4. Put the flour of your preference, egg (if you are using), salt, pepper, along with other seasonings you want in a bowl and add them. Mix to blend thoroughly. Mold into tiny patties or burgers.
5. In a big skillet, heat only 1 tbsp of coconut oil. Put 4 patties/burgers in the pan and cook 2-3

minutes on either side over medium heat. For the second half of the burgers/patties, repeat.

6. Serve with the preferred dipping sauce or low carb burger sandwich.

8. Zucchini Noodles with an Avocado Sauce

Yield: 2 – 3 servings | Prep Time: 10 Mins | Total Time: 10 Mins

Ingredients

- 1 1/4 cup basil (30 g)
- 1/3 cup water (85 ml)
- 1 zucchini
- 4 tbsp pine nuts

- 2 tbsp lemon juice
- 1 avocado
- 12 sliced cherry tomatoes

Directions

1. Using a peeler or spiralizer to produce the zucchini noodles.
2. In a mixer, mix most of the ingredients, excluding the cherry tomatoes, until creamy.
3. In a mixing dish, combine the pasta, avocado sauce, and cherry tomatoes.
4. These zucchini noodles are best fresh with avocado sauce, but you can keep them for 1 to 2 days in the fridge.

9. Avocado Chocolate Mousse

Servings: 4 | Prep Time: 5 Mins | Tot Time: 10 Mins

Ingredients

- 1 tsp. pure vanilla extract
- 1/4 cup unsweetened almond milk
- 1/8 tsp. kosher salt

- 2 large ripe avocados *(around 8 oz. each)*
- 3 tbsp. unsweetened cocoa powder
- 4 oz. chopped semisweet chocolate *or the chocolate chips (at least 60% dark, nearly 1/2 cup plus 2 tbsp.)*
- **For serving** *fresh raspberries strawberries (sliced), whipped cream or whipped coconut cream to keep vegan and chocolate shavings*
- **Optional:** 1–3 tsp. of light agave nectar *or maple syrup,*

Directions

1. In a microwave-safe dish, put the minced chocolate or the chocolate chips. Microwave in pulses of 15 seconds, stirring, and observe so that the chocolate shouldn't burn. Take it from a microwave when the chocolate is melted and stir until smooth. Put aside until just barely warm and let cool.

2. Halve and grind the avocados and scoop them into a steel blade or a high-powered blender-fitted food processor. Add cocoa powder,

melted chocolate, vanilla extract, almond milk, and salt. Blend until very creamy and smooth, stopping to scratch the bowl when desired if extra sweetness is needed, taste and add some tsp of agave. Serve as a pudding instantly, or refrigerate until cooled, 2 hours or overnight, for thickening or consistency like mousse. Topped with raspberries, chocolate shavings, and cream before serving.

10. Keto Waffles

Servings: 4 | Prep Time 5 Mins | Tot Time: 10 Mins

Ingredients

Original recipe

- 1 tbsp sweetener of choice (granulated)
- 1 tbsp applesauce can (unsweetened)
- 1 tsp coconut oil
- 1/2 tsp vanilla extract
- 1/4 cup milk of preference
- 1/4 tsp. baking powder
- 2/3 cup or 4 liquid egg whites

- 4 tbsp coconut flour sifted

Directions

1. Add your sweetener, baking powder, coconut flour, and set them aside in a deep mixing dish.

2. Add the egg whites, milk, unsweetened applesauce, and vanilla extract to a different mixing bowl and blend gently. Pour it into a dry mixture and blend until it forms a dense batter. Add the oil of your choosing and encourage the batter to sit down for 5 minutes.

3. Warm-up and gently brush your waffle iron with oil/cooking spray. When heated, add the butter, then cook until the outside is crispy, and the inside is fluffy. Repeat before you use up all the batter.

11. Low Carbohydrate Cinnamon Mug Roll Cake

Serving: 1 | Prep Time: 5 Mins | Tot Time 15-20 Mins

Ingredients

- 1/4 tsp vanilla extract
- 1/4 cup milk
- 1/2 tsp cinnamon
- 1/2 tsp cinnamon
- 1/2 tsp baking powder
- 1 tsp granulated sweetener
- 1 tbsp. granulated sweetener of choice
- 1 tbsp. coconut flour
- 1 scoop vanilla protein powder (32-34 grams)
- 1 large egg liquid egg whites)

For the glaze

- 1 tbsp coconut butter (melted)
- 1/2 tsp milk of choice
- pinch cinnamon

Directions

For the microwave option

1. Oil up with a cooking spray microwave-safe bowl and add the protein powder, cinnamon, coconut flour, baking powder, the desired sweetener, and blend well.

2. Put and blend the egg/whites into a dry mixture. If the batter is crumbly, continue adding the milk of preference until a thicker batter is made. Add the milk and vanilla extract, granulated sweetener, and extra cinnamon, then swirl over the top. Now Microwave for about 60 seconds, or before the core has just fried. Glaze on top and enjoy

For the oven option

1. Follow as above, bake for 8-15 minutes in the oven at 350 ºF, depending on the ideal consistency- Mug cake is baked if a toothpick comes out clean from the middle.

12. Carrot Cake Bites

Yield: 15 servings | Prep Time: 5 Mins | Total Time: 20 Mins

Ingredients

- 1/2 cup coconut flour
- 1/2 cup + 1 Tbsp. water
- 1/2 tsp vanilla extract
- 2 Tbsp applesauce (unsweetened)
- 1 tsp cinnamon
- 4 Tbsp Lakanto Monk Fruit Sweetener (granulated)
- 1 medium carrot (60-70g) (finely chopped or shredded)
- 4 Tbsp of reduced-fat coconut (shredded)

Directions

1. In a large mixing bowl, mix the water, applesauce, coconut flour, vanilla extract, and whisk.

2. In a dish, add the cinnamon, shredded carrots, lakanto, and whisk to mix.

3. Heat the dough for about 15 minutes.

4. In a big bowl, add shredded coconut.

5. Remove the dough from a fridge after 15 minutes and roll it into 15 equal-sized cake balls. Roll each ball until sufficiently coated with shredded coconut.

6. It can be stored in the refrigerator f0r a week.

13. Mexican-Chocolate Avocado Ice Cream

Yield: 3 servings | Prep Time: 25 Mins | Total Time: 2 hours 15 mins

Ingredients

- 1/4 - 3/4 tsp chipotle powder
- 1 15- oz. can full-fat coconut milk
- 1/3 cup Swerve Sweetener

- 1 1/2 tsp. ground cinnamon
- 1 tsp. espresso powder
- 3 oz. sugar-free dark chocolate like Lily's, (chopped)
- 1 tsp. vanilla extract
- 2 mediums of California Avocados

Directions

1. Whisk together the sweetener, espresso powder, and coconut milk in a medium saucepan at medium heat until the sweetener is dissolved. Just get it to a boil.

2. Remove and add a bar of chopped chocolate from the heat. Let sit until the chocolate has melted for 4 minutes, then whisk until perfectly smooth. Whisk in an extract of vanilla.

3. Mix the avocados, cinnamon, chocolate mixture, and chipotle in a blender or a food processor. Puree until it's smooth. Refrigerate for at least 2 hours to cool.

4. Move the mixture to an ice cream machine and swirl until the soft-serve ice cream gets

consistency (this will take less time as compared to custard-based ice creams). Serve as a soft serving or switch to a sealed jar and, for a firmer consistency, ice for another few hours.

14. Keto Broccoli Salad

Yield: 4 servings | Prep Time: 15 Mins | Total Time: 35 Mins

Ingredients

FOR THE SALAD

- kosher salt
- 3 slices of bacon (cooked and crumbled)
- 3 heads broccoli (Make bite-size pieces)
- 2 tbsp. chives (freshly chopped)
- 1/4 red onion
- 1/4 cup toasted sliced almonds
- 1/2 cup of shredded cheddar

FOR THE DRESSING

- Kosher salt
- Freshly ground black pepper

- 3 tbsp. vinegar (apple cider)
- 2/3 cup mayonnaise
- 1 tbsp. Dijon mustard

Directions

1. Put the 6 cups of salted water in a medium container or saucepan for boiling. Prepare a big bowl of ice water while waiting.

2. Place the broccoli florets in the boiling water and simmer for 1 to 2 minutes, until tender. With the slotted spoon, remove and put in the prepared ice water cup. Drain the florets in the colander while it is cold.

3. In a medium dish, whisk together the ingredients for the dressing. Season with salt & pepper to taste.

4. Mix all the ingredients for the salad in a big dish. Toss before the ingredients in the dressing are mixed and thoroughly coated. Before serving, refrigerate until fully prepared.

15. Almond Flour Waffles

Servings: 2 | Prep Time: 10 Mins | Tot Time: 20 Mins

Ingredients

- 1 tsp. kosher salt
- 1/2 cup (1 stick) butter (plus more for serving)
- 1/2 cup almond butter
- 1/4 cup granulated Swerve
- 2 cup almond flour
- 2 tsp. baking powder
- 2 tsp. pure of vanilla extract
- 4 large eggs (separated)
- Cooking spray
- Sugar-free maple syrup (for serving)

Directions

1. Preheat iron too strong for waffle. Whisk together the almond flour, baking powder, stevia, and salt in the large bowl.
2. Melt the butter & almond butter in a small microwave bowl, stir every 15 seconds. Whisk the melted butter mixture in the dry ingredients, then stir in the yolks and vanilla.

3. Beat the egg whites into firm peaks in another bowl, using a hand mixer. Fold the whites in the batter until they are mixed.

4. With the cooking spray, oiled the waffle iron, then pour half the batter in the waffle iron, then cook until slightly golden, around 5 minutes. Move to a plate and repeat for the batter that remains.

5. Include a pat of butter & maple syrup to the top.

16. Everything Keto Bagels

Yield: 8 servings | Prep Time: 15 Mins | Total Time: 35 Mins

Ingredients

- 3 tbsp. bagel seasoning
- 3 cup mozzarella cheese shredded
- 2 large eggs (1 large lightly beaten egg)
- 2 oz. cream cheese
- 2 cup almond flour
- 1 tbsp. baking powder

Directions

1. Preheat the oven to 400 °F. Line 2 parchment paper rimmed baking sheets. Stir the baking powder with the almond flour in a big bowl. Stir together the cream cheese and mozzarella cheese in a medium-sized microwave-safe bowl. Microwave until the cheese becomes melted and mixed, stirring about 30 seconds, about 2 minutes in all.

2. With an almond flour mixture, pour the cheese mixture into a bowl and then add the two eggs. Once appropriately mixed, divide the dough into eight equal servings. Roll into a ball with each section. To form a bagel shape, place your finger into the middle of each ball, then stretch. Arrange bagels on baking sheets.

3. Brush each bagel's top with beaten egg, then sprinkle all the bagel seasoning with it.

4. Bake for 20 - 24 minutes or when golden brown on the center rack. Until serving, let it cool for 10 minutes.

17. Artichoke Stuffed Peppers

Yield: 4-6 servings | Prep Time: 15 Mins | Total Time: 40 Mins

Ingredients

- 1 1/2 cup shredded mozzarella (divided)
- 1 (10-oz.) package frozen spinach (well-drained, thawed, and chopped)
- 1 (14-oz.) Can artichoke hearts (drained and chopped)
- 1/2 cup grated Parmesan
- 1/4 cup mayonnaise
- 1/4 cup sour cream
- 2 cup shredded rotisserie chicken
- 2 cloves garlic (minced)
- 4 assorted bell peppers (halved and seeded)
- 6 oz. cream cheese softened
- Chopped fresh parsley (for garnish)
- Extra-virgin olive oil (for drizzling)
- Freshly ground black pepper
- kosher salt

Directions

1. Preheat the oven to 400 ºF. Place cut side-up bell peppers on a big, rimmed baking sheet, then drizzle with the olive oil, and season with salt & pepper.

2. Place the chicken, artichoke hearts, lettuce, cream cheese, 1/2 cup of mozzarella, parmesan cheese, sour cream, garlic, and mayo in a big dish, then include more salt and pepper to season and blend until well mixed.

3. Divide the mixture of chicken between the pepper pieces, top with the leftover mozzarella, and bake for around 25 minutes until the cheese is melted and the peppers are tender.

4. Garnish and serve with parsley.

18. Best Keto Tortillas

Servings: 8 | Prep Time: 20 Mins | Tot Time: 30 Mins

Ingredients

- Almond flour
- 3 tsp. Lime juice
- 2 tsp. Xanthan gum
- 1/4 cup coconut flour
- 1/2 tsp. Kosher salt
- 1 large egg (lightly beaten)
- 1 tsp. Baking powder
- 1 tbsp. Water
- 1 cup

Directions

1. Using a food processor bowl to mix almond flour,

   xanthan gum, coconut powder, and salt. Pulse, until paired, for 5 seconds.

2. Slowly pour in the lime juice, then the egg, and then the flour mixture while the food processor operates. When the dough gets tougher, make the balls, empty it on plastic and firmly wrap it. Blend the dough in your hands for a minute or two, then put it in the fridge to cool for 10 minutes.

3. "Divide the dough into 8 small balls with a diameter of about 1 1/2". Among the two pieces of the parchment and wax paper, put one ball and roll until it's 1/8 'thick. (The diameter of the tortilla should be around 5" to 6".)

4. Over medium-high cook, heat a large iron skillet. When it is hot, include the tortilla, then cook until lightly burned. When frying one tortilla, begin rolling the next one out. Continue until you have fried and fried all the tortillas and serve instantly.

19. Zucchini Grilled Cheese

Yield: 3-4 servings | Prep Time: 40 Mins | Total Time: 40 Mins

Ingredients

- Vegetable oil (for cooking)
- kosher salt
- Freshly ground black pepper
- 2 green onions (thinly sliced)
- 2 cup shredded cheddar
- 2 cup grated zucchini
- 1/4 cup cornstarch
- 1/2 cup freshly grated Parmesan
- 1 large egg

Directions

1. With the clean kitchen towel, squeeze the remaining moisture from the zucchini. Mix the zucchini with the parmesan, green onions, egg, and cornstarch in a medium bowl. With salt and pepper, season.

2. Pour sufficient vegetable oil into a large skillet to brush the bottom of a pan. Scoop one side of the pan with around 1/4 cup of a zucchini mixture and form into a small rectangle. Repeat, on the other hand, to shape another patty.

3. Cook until both sides are softly golden, around 4 minutes per hand. Remove from the heat on paper towels to drain and repeat with the remaining mixture of zucchini. Wipe out the empty skillet.

4. Over medium heat, place two patties (zucchini) in the same skillet. Top each with the shredded cheese, then add two more patties of zucchini on top to make two sandwiches. Cook until melted, around 2 minutes per side of the cheese.

5. With the remaining ingredients, repeat. Immediately serve.

20. Bell Pepper Nachos

Servings: 6 | Prep Time: 15 Mins | Tot Time: 40 Mins

Ingredients

- Lime wedges, for serving
- Kosher salt
- Freshly ground black pepper
- 4 bell peppers (cut into small wedges)
- 2 tbsp. extra-virgin olive oil
- 1/4 tsp. garlic powder
- 1/2 tsp. ground cumin
- 1/2 tsp. chili powder
- 1/2 cup sour cream
- 1/2 cup pickled jalapeño slices
- 1 tbsp. milk (or water)
- 1 cup Pico de Gallo salsa
- 1 cup guacamole
- 1 1/2 cup Monterey Jack (shredded)
- 1 1/2 cup shredded cheddar (shredded)

Directions

1. Preheat your oven to 425 °F and cover the foil with two thin baking sheets.

2. Divide the bell peppers between sheets for baking. Place the olive oil, cumin, chili powder, and garlic powder together. With salt and pepper, season generously. Lay the wedges in a single layer, keep cut side up, on the baking sheets. Bake for about 10 minutes, until the peppers are crisp and soft.

3. With both the Monterey Jack and the cheddar, top the bell peppers. Bake for 10 minutes, until the cheese becomes bubbly.

4. Guacamole, salad, and pickled jalapeños top things off. Mix with a whip the sour cream and milk together in a small bowl and drizzle over the bell peppers. On top, pinch a lime wedge and serve with more wedges of lime.

21. Cheesy Cauli Bread

Yield: 1 serving | Prep Time: 15 Mins | Total Time: 45 Mins

Ingredients

- Pinch of red pepper flakes (crushed)
- Marinara (for dipping)

- Kosher salt
- Freshly ground black pepper
- Freshly chopped parsley
- 3 cup shredded mozzarella (divided)
- 2 large eggs
- 2 cloves garlic (minced)
- 2 tsp.
- 1/2 tsp. Dried oregano
- 1/2 cup grated parmesan
- 1 large head cauliflower

DIRECTIONS

1. Preheat the oven to 425ºF and cover the parchment with a baking sheet. Rate cauliflower in the food processor or a box grater.

2. In a large bowl, transfer the cauliflower with the eggs, oregano, 1 cup of mozzarella, garlic, Parmesan cheese, and dress with salt and pepper. Whisk once blended fully.

3. Move the dough to the baking sheet prepared and pat it into the crust. Bake for 25 minutes until they are golden and drying out.

4. Sprinkle with the leftover mozzarella, red pepper flakes (crushed), then parsley, and cook 5 to 10 more minutes before the cheese is melted.

5. Slice and serve.

22. Easy Keto Cereal

Yield: 3 servings | Prep Time: 10 Mins | Total Time: 35 Mins

Ingredients

- Cooking spray
- 2 tbsp. flax seeds
- 2 tbsp. chia seeds
- 1/4 cup sesame seeds
- 1/4 cup melted coconut oil
- 1/2 tsp. kosher salt
- 1/2 tsp. ground clove

- 1 large egg white
- 1 tsp. pure vanilla extract
- 1 cup walnuts (chopped)
- 1 cup coconut flakes (unsweetened)
- 1 cup almonds (chopped)
- 1 1/2 tsp. ground cinnamon

Directions

1. Preheat the oven to 350 °F and spray the oil on a baking sheet. Combine the almonds, walnuts, sesame seeds, coconut flakes, flax seeds, and chia seeds in a large dish. Add the garlic, vanilla, cinnamon, and salt and stir.

2. Beat the white egg until it's foamy, then stir in the granola. Then add coconut oil and now stir until it is well covered. Spread onto the prepared baking sheet then into an even layer. Now Bake for about 20 to 25 minutes or until the mixture is crispy, stirring gently halfway through. Cool it before serving.

23. Baked-Egg Avocado Boats

Servings: 4 | Prep Time: 10 Mins | Tot Time: 40 Mins

Ingredients

- Kosher salt
- Freshly ground black pepper
- Freshly chopped chives (for garnish)
- 4 large eggs
- 3 slices bacon
- 2 ripe avocados (halved and pitted)

DIRECTIONS

1. Preheat the oven to 350 ºF. Scoop about 1 tbsp of avocado; discard or store for another usage.

2. In a baking dish, put the hollowed avocados, then cut the eggs into a cup, one at a time. Move one yolk to each half of the avocado using a spoon, then spoon with as much egg white without spilling over.

3. Now, Season with salt & pepper and bake for 20 to 25 minutes, until the whites are fixed,

and the yolks are no runnier. (If avocados start to brown, cover with foil.)

4. Meanwhile, cook bacon until it is crisp (in about 8 minutes) in a large skillet over medium heat, then shift it to a paper plate (towel-lined) and chop.

5. Before serving, top the avocados with the bacon and chives.

24. Cauliflower Toast

Yield: 4-6 servings | Prep Time: 15 Mins | Total Time: 45 Mins

Ingredients

- Kosher salt
- Freshly ground black pepper
- 1/2 cup cheddar (shredded)
- 1 medium head cauliflower
- 1 large egg
- 1 tsp. Garlic powder

Directions

1. Preheat your oven to 425 ºF and cover the parchment paper with a baking sheet. Clean the cauliflower thinly and pass it to a large cup. High Microwave, 8 minutes. Drain well until the mixture is dry, with paper towels or the cheesecloth.

2. Add the egg, cheddar, and garlic powder and season with salt and pepper until mixed to the cauliflower dish.

3. On the prepared baking sheets, shape the cauliflower into the toast, then bake until golden (around 18 to 20 minutes).

4. Add the desired toppings, such as mashed avocado, bacon, a fried egg, lettuce, and tomato, to a plate and then serve.

Salads

1. Keto Egg Salad

Yield: 4 servings | Prep Time: 15 Mins | Total time: 25 Mins

INGREDIENTS

- Mayonnaise 3 tbsp.
- Lemon juice 2 tsp.
- Finely chopped chives 1 tbsp.
- Kosher salt
- Hard-boiled eggs 6
- Avocado, cubed, 1
- Cooked bacon and Lettuce (serving)
- Ground black pepper

DIRECTIONS

1. In a medium dish, mix mayonnaise, lemon juice and civet. Season to taste with salt and pepper.
2. Add the eggs and the avocado and mix gently to blend.

3. Serve with bacon and salad.

2. Grilled Chicken Salad

Servings: 4 | Prep Time: 10 Mins | Tot time: 30 Mins

Ingredients

- Boneless and skinless chicken breasts 2
- Ground coriander 1 tsp.
- Dried oregano 1 tsp.
- Kosher salt
- Ground black pepper

- Olive oil 5 tbsp.
- Red wine vinegar 4 tbsp.
- Freshly chopped parsley 1 tbsp.
- Romaine hearts, chopped, 4
- Persian cucumbers, thinly chopped, 3
- Grape or cherry tomatoes halved 1 c.
- Avocados, sliced, 2
- feta, crumbled, 4 oz.
- Pitted kalamata olives, halved, 1/2 c.

Directions

1. Heat grill to medium-high heat. Season chicken with cilantro, oregano, salt, and pepper. Grill, sealed, halfway through, before golden and no longer pink, 18 to 22 minutes. Let it rest for 5 minutes, then slice.

2. In the meantime, make the dressing. In a tiny cup, whisk olive oil, red wine vinegar and parsley and season with salt and pepper.

3. Divide cabbage, cucumbers, onions, avocado, feta, and olives into four serving bowls. Cover

with the chicken diced, then drizzle with the sauce.

3. Cobb Egg Salad

Yield: 6 servings | Prep Time: 15 Mins | Total Time: 20 Mins

Ingredients

- Mayonnaise 3 tbsp.
- Greek yogurt 3 tbsp.
- Red wine vinegar 2 tbsp.
- Kosher salt
- Ground black pepper
- Boiled eggs, 8 hard
- Bacon, cooked and crumbled, 8 strips
- 1 avocado, thinly chopped
- Crumbled blue cheese, 1/2 c.
- Cherry tomatoes halved 1/2 c.
- Freshly chopped chives 2 tbsp.

Directions

1. In a shallow dish, combine the mayonnaise, the yogurt, and the red wine vinegar. Season to taste with salt and pepper.

2. Mix the eggs, bacon, pineapple, blue cheese, and cherry tomatoes softly in a wide serving dish. Gradually add in the mayonnaise sauce, utilizing just sufficiently until the products have been finely coated, then season with salt and pepper. Marinade with chives and other toppings.

4. Loaded Cauliflower Salad

Servings: 6 | Prep Time: 10 Mins | Tot Time; 30 Mins

Ingredients

- Cauliflower, cut into florets, 1 large head
- Bacon 6 slices
- Sour cream 1/2 c.
- Mayonnaise 1/4 c.
- Lemon juice 1 tbsp.
- Garlic powder 1/2 tsp.
- Kosher salt

- Ground black pepper
- Shredded cheddar 1 1/2 c.
- Finely chopped chives 1/4 c.

DIRECTIONS

1. Bring around 1/4" of water to a boil in a large skillet. Add the cauliflower, cover the plate, and steam for around 4 minutes until tender. Drain and let it cool when you're cooking other ingredients.

2. In a wide skillet over medium heat, cook bacon until crisp, around 3 minutes per hand. Switch to a paper towel-lined dish to rinse, then chop.

3. In a big cup, stir together some heavy cream, mayonnaise, lemon juice and garlic powder. Add the cauliflower and stir softly. Dress with salt and pepper, then add in pork, cheddar, and civet. Serve hot or at room temperature.

5. Shrimpo de Gallo

Yield: 8 servings | Prep Time: 10 Mins | Total Time: 25 Mins

Ingredients

- Olive oil 1 tbsp.
- Garlic, minced, 1 clove
- Chili powder 1/4 tsp.
- Large shrimp, tails removed, 1 lb.
- Kosher salt
- Tomatoes 1 1/2 lb.
- Finely diced white onion 1/2 c.
- Finely chopped cilantro 1/2 c.
- Jalapeño peppers 2
- 1 avocado, finely chopped
- Fresh lime juice 2 tbsp.
- Tortilla chips, for serving

DIRECTIONS

1. In a large skillet heat the oil over medium-high heat. Season the shrimp with salt and add the garlic and chili powder to the skillet. Season to taste with salt. Cook, stirring until the shrimp become pink and only cooked through, around 3 minutes. Using a slotted spoon, pass the shrimp to the cutting board to cool off.

2. Break the shrimp into tiny bits and scrape into a medium dish. Add peppers, cabbage, cilantro, jalapenos, lime juice and avocado and season with salt.

3. Adjust until blended and serve with tortilla chips.

6. Chicken Salad Stuffed Avocados

Servings: 4 | Prep Time: 10 Mins | Tot Time: 10 Mins

Ingredients

- 2 avocados, pitted
- Shredded rotisserie chicken 2 c.
- Red onion, minced, 1/4 c.

- Mayonnaise 1/3 c.
- Greek yogurt 2 tbsp.
- Juice of 1 lemon
- Dijon mustard 1 1/2 tsp.
- Kosher salt
- Ground black pepper
- Chopped parsley, for garnish

Directions

1. Scoop out the attorneys, leaving a tiny border. Dice the avocat and put it aside.
2. Create chicken salad: In a big bowl, add chicken, onion, mayonnaise, yogurt, lemon juice and mustard. Fold the sliced avocado. Season to taste with salt and pepper.
3. Divide the salad into 4 avocado halves. Garnish with some parsley.

7. Parmesan Brussels Sprouts Salad

Yield: 6 servings | Prep Time: 25 Mins | Total Time: 25 Mins

Ingredients

- Olive oil 5 tbsp.
- Lemon juice 5 tbsp.
- Freshly chopped parsley 1/4 c.
- Ground black pepper
- Brussels sprouts 2 lb.
- Chopped toasted almonds 1/2 c.
- Pomegranate seeds 1/2 c.
- Shaved parmesan, for serving
- Kosher salt

Directions

1. In a medium cup, whisk olive oil, lemon juice, parsley, 2 teaspoons of salt and 1 teaspoon of pepper until mixed.
2. Add the Brussels sprouts and throw until they are fully sprayed.
3. Let stay, stirring regularly, for almost 20 minutes and 3-4 hours before serving.
4. Fold in the pomegranate seeds and almonds and garnish with shaved Parmesan before eating.

8. Shrimp Salad

Yield: 2 servings | Prep Time: 5 Mins | Total Time: 20 Mins

Ingredients

FOR SALAD

- Shrimp, peeled and deveined 1 lb.
- Olive oil 1 tbsp.
- Kosher salt
- Ground black pepper
- Red onion, finely chopped, 1/4
- Celery, finely chopped, 1 stalk
- Freshly chopped dill 2 tbsp.

FOR DRESSING

- Mayonnaise 1/2 c.
- Juice of 1 lemon
- Dijon mustard 1 tsp.

Directions

1. Preheat the oven to a temperature of 400°F. Toss shrimp with oil on a broad baking sheet and season with salt and pepper.

2. Bake until shrimp is fully opaque, for 5 to 7 minutes.

3. In a wide dish, whisk together mayonnaise, lemon juice, zest, dice, and season with salt and pepper. Add the fried shrimp, red onion, celery, and dill to the bowl and toss until incorporated.

4. Serve with bread or salad.

9. Antipasto Salad

Servings: 6 | Prep time: 10 Mins | Tot Time: 15 Mins

Ingredients

For the Salad

- Romaine hearts, chopped, 2 larges
- Salami 1/2 lb.
- Mozzarella balls, halved, 8 oz.
- Quartered artichoke hearts 1 c.
- Cherry tomatoes halved 1 c.
- Chopped pepperoncini 1 c.
- Sliced olives 1/2 c.

For the Red Wine Vinaigrette

- Olive oil 1/2 c.
- Red wine vinegar 1/4 c.
- Dijon mustard 1 tsp.
- Oregano 1/2 tsp.
- Red pepper flakes 1/4 tsp.
- Kosher salt
- Ground black pepper

Directions

1. In a big dish, add spinach, salami, mozzarella, artichokes, peppers, pepperoncini.

2. Create the vinaigrette: shake the olive oil, the vinegar, the mustard, the oregano, and the red pepper flakes in a container with a lid. Season to taste with salt and pepper.

3. Wear the vinaigrette salad and eat.

10. Greek Salad

Yield: 4 servings | Prep time: 15 Mins | Total Time: 15 Mins

Ingredients

FOR THE SALAD

- Grape or cherry tomatoes, halved, 1 pt.
- 1 cucumber
- Halved kalamata olives 1 c.
- Red onion, thinly sliced, 1/2
- Crumbled feta 3/4 c.

FOR THE DRESSING

- Red wine vinegar 2 tbsp.
- Juice of 1/2 a lemon
- Dried oregano 1 tsp.

- Kosher salt
- Ground black pepper
- Olive oil 1/4 c.

Directions

1. In a wide dish, add peppers, cucumber, olives, and red onion. Gently fold it in the feta.

2. In a small cup, mix vinegar, lemon juice and oregano and season with salt and pepper. Add the olive oil gently, whisking to mix.

3. Drizzle over the salad sauce.

11. Strawberry Spinach Salad

Yield: 4 servings | Prep Time: 15 Mins | Total Time: 20 Mins

Ingredients

- Fresh lemon juice 2 tbsp.
- Dijon mustard 1/2 tsp.
- Olive oil 1/4 c.
- Kosher salt
- Ground black pepper

- Packed baby spinach 5 c.
- Rotisserie chicken breasts 2
- Thinly sliced strawberries 2 c.
- Chopped toasted pecans 3/4 c.
- Small red onion, thinly sliced, 1/4
- Feta, crumbled, 5 oz.

Directions

1. Whisk the lemon juice with the mustard in a wide dish. Slowly add in the oil when whisking before the dressing is mixed. Season to taste with salt and pepper.
2. Add the broccoli, chicken, tomatoes, 1/2 cup of pecans and the onion to the bowl with the seasoning and toss to blend.
3. Place the salad on the plates and finish with the leftover pecans and a generous crumb of feta.

12. Caprese Salad

Yield: 4-6 servings | Prep Time: 5 Mins | Total Time: 5 Mins

Ingredients

- Fresh mozzarella 1 lb.
- Ripe tomatoes, sliced, 4 large or 6 mediums
- Basil 1 bunch
- Olive oil, for drizzling
- Freshly ground black pepper
- Flaky sea salt

Directions

1. A sheet of mozzarella and tomato slices alternately on a large pan or platter.
2. Drizzle with olive oil, season with salt and pepper.

13. Arugula Salad

Yield: 2 servings | Prep Time: 5 Mins | Total Time: 5 Mins

Ingredients

- Olive oil 6 tbsp.
- Lemon juice 2 tbsp.
- Kosher salt

- Ground black pepper
- Arugula 4 c.
- Shaved parmesan, for garnish

Directions

1. In a medium cup, whisk together olive oil and lemon juice, then season with salt and pepper.
2. In a wide dish, dress arugula gently, then finish with the parmesan.

14. Grilled Chicken Wedge Salad

Servings: 4 | Prep Time: 10 Mins | Total Time: 25 Mins

Ingredients

- Boneless and skinless chicken breasts 2
- Olive oil, plus more for drizzling, 2 tbsp.
- Kosher salt
- Ground black pepper
- Mayonnaise 1/2 c.
- Red wine vinegar 1 tbsp.
- Garlic, grated, 2 cloves
- Diced red onion 1/4 c.

- Minced chives 2 tbsp.
- Head iceberg lettuce 1 large
- 2 avocados, pitted and halved

Directions

1. Preheat the grill or stovetop toaster over extreme heat. Rinse chicken, drizzle with olive oil and season with salt and pepper. When the grill or pan is hot (almost smoking), put the chicken on the grill. Cook until the internal temperature is 165°C, 5 minutes per foot. Placed aside to rest for 2 to 3 minutes, then shredded with 2 forks.

2. In the meanwhile, plan the dressing. Put mayonnaise, red wine vinegar, olive oil, garlic, red onion, chives, salt, and pepper in a medium jar; mix well. Leave in the refrigerator until ready to serve.

3. Serve each iceberg with half a mango, a pinch of shredded chicken and a drizzle of salad dressing.

15. Cilantro-Lime Cucumber Salad

Yield: 4-6 servings | Prep Time: 5 Mins | Total Time: 8 Mins

Ingredients

- 1 jalapeno, seeded and finely sliced
- Garlic, finely minced, 2 cloves
- Fresh lime juice 3 tablespoons
- Crushed red pepper 1/4 teaspoon
- Salt 1/2 teaspoon
- Black pepper to taste
- Olive oil 3 tablespoons
- 2 cucumbers
- Minced cilantro 4 tablespoons

Directions

1. Slice the garlic and the jalapeno and add to the medium dish.

2. Add 3 tablespoons of fresh lime juice, smashed red pepper, salt and pepper to taste. Using a whisk to add 3 teaspoons of olive oil. Set it back.

3. Slice the cucumbers finely. Using a good knife or a mandolin. Add the cucumbers to the dressing and stir together.

4. Finely cut the coriander and add it to the dish. Merge them. You may either let it stay in the refrigerator and marinate for a few hours or serve immediately.

16. Greek Salmon Salad with Tahini Yogurt Dressing

Yield: 4 servings | Prep Time: 20 Mins | Total Time: 30 Mins

Ingredients

Salmon

- Skin-on wild caught salmon fillets 4 (4 oz)

- Dried dill 1/2 teaspoon
- Dried oregano 1/2 teaspoon
- Granulated garlic 1/4 teaspoon
- Kosher salt and ground black pepper to taste

Tahini Yogurt Dressing

- Plain nonfat Greek yogurt 1/2 cup
- Tahini 1 tablespoon
- Olive oil 1 1/2 teaspoons
- 1 lemon, juiced
- Ground cumin 1/4 teaspoon
- Dried dill 1/4 teaspoon
- Granulated garlic 1/4 teaspoon
- Coriander 1/4 teaspoon
- Kosher salt and ground black pepper to taste

Salad

- Chopped romaine lettuce 6 cups
- Thinly sliced red onion 1/3 cup
- Kalamata olives 1/3 cup
- Feta cheese, cubed, 2 ounces

- Diced cucumber 1 cup
- Cherry tomatoes, halved, 1/2 cup
- Olive oil 1 teaspoon
- Red wine vinegar 1 teaspoon
- Dried oregano 1/4 teaspoon
- Dried dill 1/4 teaspoon
- Kosher salt and ground black pepper to taste

Directions

1. Preheat the grill to medium heat and oil the grill. When the grill heats up, mix all the salmon spices, and use the mortar and pestle or your hands' palms to grind them. Sprinkle the salmon uniformly. Put the salmon meat side down on the grill and cook 3-5 minutes per side, depending on the thickness. Then remove it from the grill and let it rest for a few minutes before removing the skin and flaking it apart with a fork.

2. In a small dish, combine all the ingredients for the dressing and whisk until smooth. Taste for seasoning and then refrigerate until ready to eat.

3. In a medium dish, mix the red wine vinegar, oregano, olive oil, dill, salt, and pepper. Add the sliced cucumber, cherry tomatoes and red onion. Toss to merge it.

4. Add the Roman lettuce on a wide plate or in a serving dish. Cover the lettuce with a combination of cucumber, olives, feta, and salmon. Serve on the hand of the dressing.

Smoothies

1. Triple berry avocado

Ingredients

- Water 1 cup (240 ml)
- Mixed barriers ½ cup
- Avocado 100 grams
- Spinach 2 cups
- Hemp seeds 20 grams

Directions

Combine all the ingredients well until smooth and serve it.

2. Chocolate Peanut (Butter)

Ingredients

- Almond milk 1 cup
- Creamy peanut butter 2 tablespoons
- Cocoa powder 1 tablespoon
- Heavy cream ¼ cup
- Ice 1 cup

Directions

Combine all the ingredients well until smooth and serve it.

3. Strawberry zucchini chia

Ingredients

- Water 1 cup (240 ml)
- Frozen strawberries 1/2 cup (110 grams)
- Chopped zucchini 1 cup (124 grams)
- Chia seeds 3 tablespoons (41 grams)

Directions

Combine all the ingredients well until smooth and serve it.

4. Coconut blackberry mint

Ingredients

- Unsweetened full-fat coconut milk 1/2 cup
- Frozen blackberries 1/2 cup
- Shredded coconut 2 tablespoons
- Mint leaves 5–10

Directions

Combine all the ingredients well until smooth and serve it.

5. Lemon cucumber green smoothie

Ingredients

- Water 1/2 cup
- Ice 1/2 cup
- Sliced cucumber 1 cup
- Spinach or kale 1 cup
- Lemon juice 1 tablespoon (30 ml) of
- Milled flax seeds 2 tablespoons

Directions

Combine all the ingredients well until smooth and serve it.

6. Cinnamon raspberry breakfast smoothie

Ingredients

- Unsweetened almond milk 1 cup
- Frozen raspberries 1/2 cup
- Spinach or kale 1 cup
- Almond butter 2 tablespoons
- Cinnamon 1/8 teaspoon

Directions

Combine all the ingredients well until smooth and serve it.

7. Strawberries and cream smoothie

Ingredients

- Water 1/2 cup
- Frozen strawberries 1/2 cup
- Heavy cream 1/2 cup

Directions

Combine all the ingredients well until smooth and serve it.

8. Chocolate cauliflower breakfast smoothie

Ingredients

- Unsweetened almond or coconut milk 1 cup
- Frozen cauliflower florets 1 cup
- Unsweetened cocoa powder 1.5 tablespoons
- Hemp seeds 3 tablespoons
- cacao nibs 1 tablespoon
- A pinch of sea salt

Directions

Combine all the ingredients well until smooth and serve it.

9. Pumpkin spice smoothie

Ingredients

- Unsweetened coconut 1/2 cup
- Pumpkin purée 1/2 cup
- Almond butter 2 tablespoons
- Pumpkin pie spice 1/4 teaspoon of
- Ice 1/2 cup

- A pinch of salt

Directions

Combine all the ingredients well until smooth and serve it.

10. Lime pie smoothie

Ingredients

- Water 1 cup
- Unsweetened almond milk 1/2 cup
- raw cashews 1/4 cup
- Spinach 1 cup
- Shredded coconut 2 tablespoons
- Lime juice 2 tablespoons

Directions

Combine all the ingredients well until smooth and serve it.

Desserts

1. Keto Sugar-Free Cheesecake

Yields:8 – 10 Servings | Prep time: 15 mins | Total time:8 hours

Ingredients

- Almond flour 1/2 c.
- Coconut flour 1/2 c.
- Shredded coconut 1/4 c.
- (1 stick) butter melted 1/2 c.
- Blocks cream cheese, softened to room temperature 8-oz.
- Sour cream, at room temperature 16 oz.
- Stevia 1 tbsp.
- Pure vanilla extracts 2 tsp.
- Eggs 3, at room temperature
- For serving, sliced strawberries

Directions

1. Heat oven at 300°F. Make the crust: grease an eight/ nine spring shape pan, & cover bottom &

edges with the foil. In med bowl, mix butter & flours. Press crust in the bottom & little up sides of prepared pan. Put the pan in the fridge, whereas you make filling.

2. Make the filling: In a bowl, beat sour cream & cream cheese together, then beat in vanilla & stevia. Mix eggs one at a time, mixing every addition afterward. Spread filling equally on the crust.

3. Put the cheesecake in a roasting pan & set it on the oven of the middle rack. Cautiously put adequate boiling water in the roasting pan to come middle upsides of the spring shape pan. Bake at least one hour to one hour twenty minutes until it lightly jiggles in the middle. Turn the oven off, then leave the cake in the oven with the door a little bit open to cool gradually for at least an hour.

4. Take away pan from the water bath & take off the foil; let chill in the fridge for a minimum of 5 hours/ overnight. Slice & garnish with the strawberries.

2. Keto Chocolate Chip Cookies

Yields:18 Servings | Prep time: 15 mins | Total time:30 mins

Ingredients

- Eggs 2
- One stick melted butter 1/2 c.
- Heavy cream 2 tbsp.
- Pure vanilla extracts 2 tsp.
- Almond flour 2 3/4 c.
- Kosher salt 1/4 tsp.
- Dark chocolate chips 3/4 c.
- Granulated sugar 1/4 c.
- Cooking spray

Directions

1. Preheat oven at 350°F. In a large bowl, beat egg with butter, vanilla & heavy cream. Mix in salt, almond flour & swerve.

2. Wrinkle chocolate chips in cookie batter. Make batter into one " ball & arrange three " separately on the parchment-lined sheets of baking. Compress balls with the bottom of the glass that has been slightly greased with the cooking spray.

3. Bake till cookies is slightly golden, around seventeen to nineteen minutes.

3. Keto Chocolate Cake

Yields:12 Servings | Prep time 15 mins | Total time:1 hr. 30 mins

Ingredients

For the cake

- Cooking spray
- Almond flour 1 1/2 c.
- Unsweetened cocoa powder 2/3 c.
- Coconut flour 3/4 c.

- Flaxseed meal 1/4 c.
- Baking powder 2 tsp.
- Baking soda 2 tsp.
- Kosher salt 1 tsp.
- Keto-friendly granulated sugar 3/4 cup
- Eggs 4
- Pure vanilla extracts 1 tsp.
- One stick butter softened 1/2 cup
- Almond milk 1 cup
- Strong brewed coffee 1/3 c.

For the buttercream

- Blocks of cream cheese softened 8-oz.
- (1 stick) butter softened 1/2 cup
- Unsweetened cocoa powder 1/2 cup
- Coconut flour 1/2 cup
- Instant coffee powder 1/4 tsp.
- Keto-friendly powdered sugar 3/4 cup
- Heavy cream 3/4 cup
- Pinch kosher salt

Directions

1. Preheat oven at 350° & line 2 eight" pans with the parchment & grease with the cooking spray. In a large bowl, salt, beat together cocoa powder, flaxseed meal, baking soda, almond flour, coconut flour & baking powder.

2. Use a hand mixer in the additional large bowl, beat swerve & butter together till fluffy & light. Put eggs, one at a time; after that, mix vanilla. Put dry ingredients & mix till combined, then mix in the milk & coffee.

3. Divide the batter b/w prepared pans & bake till toothpick is inserted into middle & comes out clean, twenty-eight minutes. Ultimately allow it to cool.

4. For the frosting: in a bowl, with the hand mixer, beat butter & cream cheese together till smooth. Put cocoa powder, instant coffee, swerve & coconut flour, & beat till no lumps are left. Put cream & pinch of the salt & beat till combined.

5. Place the cake layer on the serving platter/ cake stand; after that, spread a thick layer of buttercream on the top. Again, do it with the

remaining layers; after that, frost the sides of the cake.

6. Keep refrigerated till prepared to serve

4. Keto Chocolate Mug Cake

Yields:1 Servings | Prep time: 5 mins | Total time: 5 mins

Ingredients

- Butter 2 tbsp.
- Almond flour 1/4 c.
- Cocoa powder 2 tbsp.
- Egg 1, beaten
- Keto-friendly chocolate chips 2 tbsp.
- Granulated swerve 2 tbsp.
- Baking powder 1/2 tsp.
- Pinch kosher salt
- whipped cream 1/4 c

Directions

1. Put butter in the microwave-safe mug & heat till melt, thirty seconds. Put remaining ingredients

excluding whipped cream & stir till thoroughly combined. Cook for forty-five seconds to one minute/ till cake is fully set, but still fudgy.

2. Top with the whipped cream previously serving.

5. Keto Ice Cream

Yields:8 Servings | Prep time: 5 mins | Total time:8 hours 15 mins

Ingredients

- Cans coconut milk 15-oz
- Heavy cream 2 c.
- Swerve confectioner's sweetener 1/4 c.
- Pure vanilla extracts 1 tsp.
- Pinch kosher salt

Directions

1. Cool the coconut milk in the fridge for a minimum of three hours, preferably overnight.

2. For whipped coconut: spoon the coconut cream into a bowl, leaving the liquid in the can, & use the hand mixer to whisk the coconut cream till creamy. Set apart.

3. For the whipped cream, use a hand mixer and beat the heavy cream until soft peaks are formed in the separate bowl. Beat in the vanilla & sweetener.

4. Fold the whipped coconut in the whipped cream; after that, transfer the combination into the loaf pan.

5. Freeze till solid, around five hours.

6. Keto Hot Chocolate

Yields:1 Servings | Prep time: 5 mins | Total time: 10 mins

Ingredients

- Unsweetened cocoa powder 2 tbsp, more for garnish
- Keto-friendly sugar 2 1/2 tsp, such as swerve
- Water 1 1/4 c.
- Heavy cream 1/4 c.
- Pure vanilla extracts 1/4 tsp.
- For serving, whipped cream

Directions

1. In a small saucepan on med-low heat, beat together swerve & cocoa, around two tablespoons of water till smooth & dissolved. Raise the heat to med, put remaining cream & water, & whisk irregularly till hot.
2. Mix in vanilla; after that, pour into the mug. Serve with the whipped cream & dusting of the cocoa powder.

7. Keto Pumpkin Cheesecake

Yields: 16 Servings | Prep time: 10 mins | Total time: 7 hours 30 mins

Ingredients

For the crust

- Almond flour 1 1/2 c.
- Coconut flour 1/4 c.
- Granulated swerve 2 tbsp.
- Cinnamon 1/2 tsp.
- Kosher salt 1/4 tsp.
- Butter 7 tbsp, melted

For the filling

- Blocks cream cheese 8-oz, softened
- Brown sugar swerves 1/2 c.
- Pumpkin purée 1 c.
- Eggs 3
- Pure vanilla extracts 1 tsp.
- Cinnamon 1 tsp.
- Ground ginger 1/2 tsp.
- Kosher salt 1/4 tsp.
- Whipped cream, for garnish
- Chopped toasted pecans for garnish

Directions

1. Preheat oven at 350°F. In the bowl, mix coconut flour, almond flour, cinnamon, swerve & salt. Put melted butter & mix till thoroughly combined. Press crust into an eight" spring shape pan in an equal layer little up of sides. Bake till slightly golden, ten to fifteen minutes.

2. Reduce the oven to 325°F. In the bowl, beat the cream cheese & swerve together till fluffy & light. Put pumpkin purée & beat till no lumps are left. Put eggs one at a time & beat till nicely combined. Put vanilla, ginger, cinnamon & salt. Put the batter on the top of the crust & smooth top with the offset spatula.

3. Wrap the pan bottom in aluminum foil & place in the roasting pan. Put in adequate boiled water to come up the middle in the baking pan.

4. Bake till the middle of the cheesecake only slightly jiggles, around one hour. Turn off the heat, prop open the oven door, & allow cheesecake to cool in the oven, one hour.

5. Take away foil & refrigerate cheesecake till thoroughly chilled, at least five hours & up to the whole night.

6. Serve with a dollop of toasted pecans & whipped cream.

8. Keto Pumpkin Pie

Yields:16 Servings | Prep time: 15 mins | Total time:3 hours 30 mins

Ingredients

For the crust

- Almond flour 1 1/2 c.
- Coconut flour 3 tbsp.
- Baking powder 1/4 tsp.
- Kosher salt 1/4 tsp.
- Butter 4 tbsp, melted
- Egg 1, beaten

For the filling

- Can pumpkin puree 15-oz.
- Heavy cream 1 cup
- Brown sugar 1/2 cup
- Eggs 3, beaten
- Ground cinnamon 1 tsp.

- Ground ginger 1/2 tsp.
- Ground nutmeg 1/4 tsp.
- Ground cloves 1/4 tsp.
- Kosher salt 1/4 tsp.
- Pure vanilla extracts 1 tsp.
- For serving, whipped cream

Directions

1. Preheat the oven to 350°F. In a bowl, beat together coconut flour, almond flour, salt & baking powder. Put melted butter & egg & mix till a dough shape. Press the dough equally into a nine" pie plate; after that, use a fork to stab holes all over the crust.
2. Bake till slightly golden, ten minutes.
3. In the large bowl, beat together brown sugar, cream, pumpkin, eggs, vanilla & spices till smooth. Put pumpkin combination into the par-baked crust.
4. Bake till filling is slightly jiggly in middle & crust is golden, forty-five to fifty minutes.

5. The oven is turn off & prop the door open. Allow pie to cool in the oven for one hour; after that, refrigerate until prepared to serve.

6. Serve with the whipped cream, if wanted.

9. Keto Peanut Butter Cookies

Yields:22 Servings | Prep time: 5 mins | Total time:1 hr. 30 mins

Ingredients

- Melted, smooth unsweetened peanut butter 1 1/2 c.
- Coconut flour 1 c.
- Brown sugar 1/4 c.
- Pure vanilla extracts 1 tsp.
- Pinch kosher salt
- Dark chocolate chips 2 cups
- Coconut oil 1 tbsp.

Directions

1. In a bowl, mix coconut flour, peanut butter, sugar, salt & vanilla. Mix until even.

2. Line baking sheet with baking release paper. Use cookie scoop, shape mixture into rounds, then press down slightly to flatten & place on the baking sheet. Freeze till firm, around one hour.

3. In a bowl, beat together melted chocolate & coconut oil.

4. Use a fork, dip the peanut butter in chocolate till completely coated & return to the baking sheet. Sprinkle with additional peanut butter, freeze till chocolate sets, around ten minutes.

5. Serve cold. Store any remaining in the freezer.

10. Magic Keto Cookies

Servings:15 | Prep time: 10 mins | Tot time: 35 mins

Ingredients

- Coconut oil 1/4 c.
- Butter 3 tbsp, softened
- Granulated 3 tbsp, swerve sweetener
- Kosher salt 1/2 tsp.
- Egg yolks 4
- Sugar-free dark chocolate chips 1 c, such as lily's

- Coconut flakes 1 c.
- Roughly chopped walnuts 3/4 c.

Directions

1. Preheat the oven at 350°F & line the baking sheet with baking release paper. In a bowl, mix butter, coconut oil, salt, egg yolks & sweetener. Combine in walnuts, coconut & chips.

2. Drop your batter by a spoonful onto the organized baking sheet & bake till golden fifteen minutes.

11. Chocolate Keto Cookies

Yields: 11 Servings | Prep time: 10 mins | Total time: 25 mins

Ingredients

- Butter, 2 1/2 tbsp.
- Keto chocolate chips 3 tbsp.
- Egg 1
- Pure vanilla extracts 1 tsp.
- Blanched almond flour 2/3 c.

- Confectioners swerve 1/3 c.
- Dark cocoa powder 3 1/2 tbsp.
- Baking powder 1/2 tsp.
- Pinch kosher salt

Directions

1. Preheat the oven to 325°F. In a med bowl, put butter & half chocolate chips. Microwave for fifteen to thirty seconds adequate time to lightly melt the chocolate & butter. Combine the two till chocolate sauce is made.

2. In a small dish, add & whisk egg till yolk mixes with whites. Once it fixes, put egg & vanilla extract into bowl with chocolate sauce. Combine it again.

3. Put remaining dry ingredients – save some chocolate chips to the top cookies. Combine the ball of chocolate cookie dough shapes.

4. Use cookie scoop/ a tablespoon to shape eleven evenly shaped cookies. Put cookies on the cookie sheet lined with bakery release paper & top every cookie with leftover chocolate chips. Flatten every cookie with a spoon/ spatula.

5. Bake at least eight to ten minutes. They must be well soft & when coming out of the oven but don't concern, it is normal.

6. Allow the cookies to cool down on the baking sheet. As it cool, they will adjust & firm up.

7. When they cool down, enjoy & store the reaming's in an airtight container in the fridge.

12. Keto Walnut Snowballs

Servings: 15 | Prep time: 10 mins | Total time: 1 hr. 5 mins

Ingredients

- Melted 1/2 c. Butter 1 stick
- Egg 1

- Liquid stevia 50 drops around 1/4 tsp.
- Pure vanilla extracts 1/2 tsp.
- Walnuts 1 c.
- Coconut flour 1/2 c., plus one to two tbsp. Additional for rolling
- Confectioners swerve 1/2 c

Directions

1. Preheat oven at 300°F & line baking sheet with the parchment paper. Mix melted butter, stevia, egg & vanilla extract in a bowl & set aside.

2. Put walnuts into the food processor & pulse till the ground. Put walnut flour into a bowl & put coconut flour & 1/4 cup swerve & pulse till mixed.

3. In 2 parts, put the dry mixture to wet & beat to combine. At that point, the dough must be soft but firm adequate to shape into the balls by hand without it penetrating to palms. If right uniformity is not achieved, put one to two tablespoons of extra coconut flour & combine.

4. Make fifteen evenly sized balls & arrange them on the prepared baking sheet.

5. Bake for thirty minutes.

6. Let to cool for five minutes, & then roll balls in the rest of 1/4 cup swerve.

7. Put back on parchment paper & let to complete cool, additional twenty to thirty minutes, before consumption.

13. Keto Pecan Crescents

Yields:20 Servings | Prep time: 20 mins | Total time:1 hr. 5 mins

Ingredients

For the cookies

- Almond flour 2 c.
- Finely chopped pecans 1 c.
- Coconut flour 2 tbsp.
- Baking powder 1/2 tsp.
- Kosher salt 1/4 tsp.
- Butter 1/2 c, softened one stick
- Swerve brown sugar 2/3 c./regular swerve &2 tsp. Yukon syrup

- Egg 1
- Pure vanilla extracts 1/2 tsp.

For the vanilla glaze

- Powdered Swerve sweetener 2/3 c. /powdered erythritol
- Heavy cream six to eight tbsp
- Pure vanilla extracts 1/2 tsp.

Directions

For the cookies

1. Preheat the oven at 325°F & line two baking sheets with the parchment paper. In a bowl, beat together chopped pecans, almond flour, coconut flour, salt & baking powder.

2. In a bowl, beat the butter with swerving till fluffy & light, around two minutes. Whisk in egg & vanilla extract. Whisk in almond flour combination till dough originates together.

3. Form dough into 3/4", afterward that roll between the palms & shape into crescents. Put on ready baking sheets.

4. Bake fifteen to eighteen minutes/ until slightly golden brown. Not be firm to touch, but then firm as they cool. Cool one-sheets.

For the glaze

1. Beat powdered swerve with the 1/4 cup of cream &vanilla extract till smooth. Put one tablespoon additional cream at a time till thin but spreadable uniformity is attained.

2. Put on cooled cookies & decorate as wanted.

3. Otherwise, just roll cookies in the powdered sweetener.

14. Keto Frosty

Servings: 4 | Prep time: 10 mins | Tot time: 45 mins

Ingredients

- Unsweetened cocoa powder 2 tbsp.
- Sugar sweetener 3 tbsp
- Pinch kosher salt
- Heavy whipping cream 1 1/2 c.
- Pure vanilla extracts 1 tsp.

Directions

1. In a large bowl, mix cream, vanilla, cocoa, sweetener & salt. Use hand mixer/ the beater attachment of beat mixer, stand mixer, till stiff peaks shape. Scoop mixture into the Ziploc bag & freeze for thirty to thirty-five minutes, till just frozen.

2. Cut the tip off corner of the Ziplock bag & pipe it into the serving dishes.

15. Keto Peanut Butter Sandies

Yields:15 Servings | prep time: 15 mins | Total time: 40 mins

Ingredients

- Butter 4 tbsp, softened
- Granulated swerve 1/3 c.
- Natural unsweetened peanut butter 1/2 c.
- Large egg yolk 1
- Almond flour 1/2 c.
- Coconut flour 1 tbsp.
- Kosher salt 1/4 tsp, additional for sprinkling

- For the topping, finely chopped pecans 2 tbsp.

Directions

1. Preheat oven at 350° & line baking sheet with the parchment paper.

2. Use the beater & mix cream, swerve & butter till fluffy & light in a bowl. Put in peanut butter & whisk till fully incorporated. Beat in yolk till thoroughly combined. Fold in the coconut flour, almond flour & salt & mix up until dough somewhat stiffens.

3. Use a cookie scoop, scoop the dough onto a ready sheet one" apart. Drizzle cookies with additional salt & pecans.

4. Bake till bottoms is golden, around eleven minutes.

5. Cool fully before serving

16. Keto Brownies

Yields: 16 Servings | Prep time: 15 Mins | Total time: 1hr 25 Mins

Ingredients

- Eggs 4
- Ripe avocados 2
- Melted butter 1/2 c
- Peanut butter (unsweetened) 6 tbsp
- Baking soda 2 tsp
- Granulated sugar 2/3 c
- Unsweetened cocoa powder 2/3 c
- Pure vanilla extracts 2 tsp.
- Kosher salt 1/2 tsp
- Flaky sea salt

Directions

1. Oven preheated to 350 degrees F and lined the 8"-x-8" square pan with bakery release paper.

In a blender, mix all the ingredients except the flaky sea salt & blend till smooth.

2. Move batter to the prepared cooking pan & smooth the top with the spatula. If using, Top it with flaky sea salt.

3. Cook till brownies become soft, 25-30 mins.

4. Allow it to cool for 25- 30 mins before slicing & serving.

17. Chocolate Keto Protein Shake

Yields:1 Servings | Prep time:5 Mins | Total time:5 mins

Ingredients

- Almond milk 3/4 c.
- Ice 1/2 c.
- Cocoa powder 2 tbsp.
- Sugar 2-3 tbsp
- Almond butter 2 tbsp.
- Chia seeds 1 tbsp.
- Hemp seeds 2 tbsp

- Pure vanilla extract 1/2 tbsp
- Kosher salt

Directions

1. In the blender, mix all ingredients & blend till smooth. Place into the glass & garnish it with chia & hemp seeds.

18. Keto Double Chocolate Muffins

Yields:1 dozen Servings | Prep time:10 Mins | Total time:25 mins

Ingredients

- Almond flour 2 c
- Unsweetened cocoa powder 3/4 c
- Swerve sweetener 1/4 c
- Baking powder 1 1/2 tsp
- Kosher salt 1 tsp.
- Melted butter 1 c.
- Eggs 3
- Pure vanilla extract 1 tsp
- Dark chocolate chips sugar-free 1 c

Directions

1. Oven Preheated to 350 degrees F & line the muffin tin with the liners. In the bowl, stir together cocoa powder, almond flour, Swerve, baking powder, & salt. Put the melted butter, vanilla & eggs, then stir till combined.

2. Fold in the chips of chocolate.

3. Split batter b/w muffin liners & bake till the toothpick inserted into the center comes out clean, twelve mins.

19. Cookie Dough Keto Fat Bombs

Yields: 30 Servings | Prep time: 5 Mins | Total time: 1hr 5 Mins

Ingredients

- Softened butter 1/2 c
- Confectioners' sugar (Keto friendly) 1/3 c.
- Pure vanilla extract 1/2 tsp
- Kosher salt 1/2 tsp
- Almond flour 2 c
- Dark chocolate chips (Keto friendly) 2/3 c

Directions

1. Beat butter till light & fluffy in the bowl by using a hand mixer. Put sugar, salt & vanilla, then beat till combined.
2. Gradually beat in the almond flour till no dry spots left, folding in the chocolate chips. Wrap your bowl & put it in the refrigerator, 15- 20 mins.
3. Use the cookie scoop to scoop the dough into the balls.

20. Keto Avocado Pops

Yields:10 Servings | Prep time:5 Mins |Total time:6 hours 10 Mins

Ingredients

- Ripe avocados 3
- Lime Juice 1/3 cup
- Swerve 3 tbsp
- Coconut milk 3/4 c
- Coconut oil 1 tbsp
- Chocolate (keto-friendly) 1 c

Directions

1. In the blender, mix avocados with juice of the lime, Swerve, & coconut milk. Grind till smooth & place into the popsicle mold.
2. Freeze for six hours, till firm.
3. In the bowl, mix chocolate chips & coconut oil. Microwave till melted; after this, allow it to cool at room temp. Dip the freeze pops in the chocolate & serve.

21. Keto Chocolate Truffles

Servings: 15 | prep time:10 Mins | Tot time:30 Mins

Ingredients

- Melted dark chocolate chips 1 c
- Mashed avocado one med
- Vanilla extract 1 tsp
- Kosher salt 1/4 tsp
- Cocoa powder 1/4 c

Directions

1. In the bowl, mix the melted chocolate with vanilla, salt & avocado. Whisk together till smooth & combined thoroughly. Put it in the refrigerator for 15- 20 mins.

2. Once the chocolate combination has stiffened, use the cookie scoop to scoop around one tbsp chocolate combination. Roll the chocolate into your hand palm till round; after this, roll in cocoa powder.

22. Carrot Cake Keto Balls

Yields:16 Servings | Prep time:5 Mins | Total time:15 Mins

Ingredients

- Softened block cream cheese 8-oz

- Coconut flour 3/4 c
- Stevia 1 tsp.
- Pure vanilla extract 1/2 tsp
- Cinnamon 1 tsp
- Ground nutmeg 1/4 tsp.
- Grated carrots 1 c
- Chopped pecans 1/2 c
- (unsweetened) shredded coconut 1 c

Directions

1. Whisk together the coconut flour, cream cheese, stevia, cinnamon, nutmeg & vanilla in the bowl. Fold in pecans & carrots.
2. Roll into sixteen balls, after which roll in the shredded coconut & serve.

23. Chocolate Blueberry Clusters

Yield:15 servings | Prep time:10-15 Mins | Total time:25 Mins

Ingredients

- Melted semisweet chocolate chips 1 1/2 c

- Coconut oil 1 tbsp
- Blueberries 2 c
- Flaky sea salt

Directions

1. Line the cookie sheet with bakery release paper. In the bowl, combine melted chocolate with the coconut oil.
2. Spoon the tiny chocolate dollop on parchment & top it with 4- 5 blueberries. Sprinkle chocolate on blueberries and season with sea salt.
3. Freeze for ten minutes & Serve.

24. Keto Fat Bombs

Yields:16 Servings | prep time:5 mins | total time:30 mins

Ingredients

- Cream cheese 8 oz
- Peanut butter (keto-friendly) 1/2 c
- Coconut oil 1/4 c plus 2 tbsp
- Kosher salt 1/4 tsp

- Dark chocolate chips (keto-friendly) 1/2 c

Directions

1. Line the small cookie sheet with bakery release paper. In the bowl, mix peanut butter, cream cheese, coconut oil ¼ cup, & salt. Use the hand mixer to beat the mixture till combined thoroughly, around two minutes. Put the bowl in the freezer for 10- 15 mins.

2. Once the mixture of peanut butter has hardened, use the cookie scoop to make tbsp-sized balls. Put in the refrigerator for five mins.

3. Therefore, make the drizzle of chocolate: mix chocolate chips & leftover coconut oil in the microwave-safe bowl & microwave for thirty seconds till melted fully. Sprinkle over the peanut butter balls & put back in the refrigerator for five mins.

4. Keep it covered in the refrigerator if you want to store it.

25. Chocolate Covered Strawberry Cubes

Servings: 15 | Prep Time: 10 Mins | Tot time: 4 hours 10 Mins

Ingredients

- Chocolate chips 2 c
- Coconut oil 2 tbsp
- Fresh strawberries 16

Directions

1. In the bowl, whisk together the melted chocolate chips & coconut oil.
2. Spoon the layer of the mixture of chocolate into the bottom of every ice cube mold, after this top every with the strawberry, stem side-up. Spoon leftover chocolate combination on strawberries.
3. Freeze till chocolate becomes solid, 4- 5 hours.

26. Keto Brownie Bombs

Yields: 18 Servings | Prep Time: 5 Mins | Total Time: 30 Mins

Ingredients

- Block cream cheese 8-oz
- Swerve confectioner's sugar 1/3 c
- Coconut oil 1/4 c
- Unsweetened cocoa powder 1/4 c.
- Dark chocolate chips 2/3 c

Directions

1. In the bowl, beat swerve, cream cheese, coconut oil, & cocoa powder together. After this, fold in chocolate chips.
2. Use the cookie scoop to shape the mixture into the balls & put on the parchment-lined cookie sheet.
3. Put in the freezer for 20 mins & serve.

27. Sugar-Free Low Carb Keto Avocado Brownies

Yields:12 Servings | Prep Time10 minutes | Total Time40 minutes

Ingredients

- Mashed avocado 1 cup
- Vanilla 1/2 tsp
- Cocoa powder 4 tbsp
- Refined coconut oil 3 tbsp
- Eggs 2
- Melted lily's chocolate chips 1/2 cup

Dry Ingredients

- Blanched almond flour 3/4 cup
- Baking soda 1/4 tsp
- Baking powder 1 tsp
- Salt 1/4 tsp

- Erythritol 1/4 cup
- Stevia powder 1 tsp

Directions

1. Oven preheated to 350 degrees F.
2. In the other bowl, combine the dry ingredients & stir together.
3. Peel your avocados. Put in the food processor & process till smooth.
4. Put every wet ingredient to your food processor, one at a time, & process for some seconds till all the wet ingredients are added to your food processor.
5. Put the dry ingredients in your food processor & mix till combined.
6. Put a piece of bakery release paper on the 30x20cm baking dish & place the batter into it. Spoon equally & put in the heated oven. Bake it for thirty minutes, or till a toothpick inserted in the center comes out half clean.
7. Please remove it from the oven, allow it to cool fully before slicing it into twelve pieces.

29. Keto Peanut Butter Cheesecake Bites

Yields: 2-4 Servings | Prep time:10 mins |Total time:30 Mins

Ingredients

- Softened cream cheese 8 oz
- Powdered erythritol 1/4 cup
- Vanilla extract 1 tsp
- Heavy whipping cream 1/4 cup
- Peanut butter 1/4 cup
- Sugar-Free Lily's chocolate 3/4 cup
- Coconut oil 2 tsp

Directions

1. Combine erythritol, heavy whipping cream & cream cheese till smooth
2. Mix in the peanut butter & vanilla extract till combined thoroughly, set aside
3. Melt the chocolate & mix it with coconut oil
4. Brush the cups of silicones with a mixture of chocolate & put in the freezer for five mins

5. Do the previous step again & freeze for ten mins

6. Into the cup, Put the couple spoonsful of cheesecake fluff & freeze it for fifteen mins

7. Top the cups with the chocolate to cover cheesecake fluff

8. Freeze it for twenty mins.

30. Paleo Vegan Coconut Crack Bars - Healthy 3 Ingredient - No Bake

Yields:20 Servings | Prep Time:2 mins |Total Time:5 mins

Ingredients

- Unsweetened shredded coconut flakes 3 cups
- Melted coconut oil 1 cup
- Maple syrup 1/4 cup

Directions

1. Line the 8 x 8-inch pan with bakery release paper & set aside.

2. In the mixing bowl, put the shredded coconut (unsweetened). Put the melted coconut oil &

monk fruit sweetened maple syrup & mix till a thick batter remains.

3. Put the mixture of coconut crack bar into a lined pan. Slightly wet the hands & press it firmly into the place. Refrigerate till firm. Cut into the bars & enjoy.

31. Healthy Minute Low Carb Cinnamon Roll Mug Cake

Yields:1 Servings | Prep Time: 5 Mins | Total Time: 10-15 Mins

Ingredients

- Vanilla protein powder one scoop
- Baking powder 1/2 tsp
- Coconut flour 1 T
- Cinnamon 1/2 tsp
- Granulated sweetener 1 T
- Egg 1
- Milk 1/4 cup
- Vanilla extract 1/4 tsp
- Granulated sweetener 1 tsp

- Cinnamon 1/2 tsp

For the glaze

- Melted coconut butter 1 T
- Milk 1/2 tsp
- Cinnamon pinch

Directions

For the microwave option

1. Oil the microwave-safe bowl with your cooking spray & add the baking powder, protein powder, cinnamon, coconut flour & sweetener, then mix well.

2. Put the egg whites & mix into the dry combination. Put the milk & vanilla extract- If the batter is too crumbly, add the milk until the very thick batter is created. Add granulated sweetener & additional cinnamon, then swirl on the top. Microwave it for sixty seconds. Top it with glaze & serve.

For the oven option

Follow as above but bake in an oven over 350 F for 8 to 15 mins.

32. Homemade Sugar-Free Nutella

Servings : 6 | Prep Time: 10 minutes | Tot Time: 20 minutes

Ingredients

- Toasted & husked hazelnuts 3/4 cup
- Melted coconut oil 2-3 tbsp
- Cocoa powder 2 tbsp
- Powdered Swerve Sweetener 2 tbsp
- Vanilla extract 1/2 tsp
- Pinch salt

Directions

1. In the food processor, blend hazelnuts till finely ground.

2. Put two tbsp of oil & continue to blend till nuts smooth out into the butter. Put the leftover ingredients & blend till well.

COOKING CONVERSION CHART

Measurement

CUP	ONCES	MILLILITERS	TABLESPOONS
8 cup	64 oz	1895 ml	128
6 cup	48 oz	1420 ml	96
5 cup	40 oz	1180 ml	80
4 cup	32 oz	960 ml	64
2 cup	16 oz	480 ml	32
1 cup	8 oz	240 ml	16
3/4 cup	6 oz	177 ml	12
2/3 cup	5 oz	158 ml	11
1/2 cup	4 oz	118 ml	8
3/8 cup	3 oz	90 ml	6
1/3 cup	2.5 oz	79 ml	5.5
1/4 cup	2 oz	59 ml	4
1/8 cup	1 oz	30 ml	3
1/16 cup	1/2 oz	15 ml	1

Temperature

FAHRENHEIT	CELSIUS
100 °F	37 °C
150 °F	65 °C
200 °F	93 °C
250 °F	121 °C
300 °F	150 °C
325 °F	160 °C
350 °F	180 °C
375 °F	190 °C
400 °F	200 °C
425 °F	220 °C
450 °F	230 °C
500 °F	260 °C
525 °F	274 °C
550 °F	288 °C

Weight

IMPERIAL	METRIC
1/2 oz	15 g
1 oz	29 g
2 oz	57 g
3 oz	85 g
4 oz	113 g
5 oz	141 g
6 oz	170 g
8 oz	227 g
10 oz	283 g
12 oz	340 g
13 oz	369 g
14 oz	397 g
15 oz	425 g
1 lb	453 g

Conclusion

An answer is provided as to why a ketogenic diet is so popular: it works, and weight reduction is merely only the beginning. Studies have shown that this diet enhances energy levels, stabilizes mood, controls sugar in the blood, boosts cholesterol, lowers blood pressure, and more. For intractable epilepsy, the keto diet promises safe and reasonably balanced treatment. Despite its long history, though, much remains uncertain about the diet, including its modes of operation, the right therapy, and the broad reach of its applicability.

Diet experiments provide useful insight into the origins of seizures and epilepsy themselves, as well as the required alternative therapies. However, the diet's inadequate execution may have significant health effects and may not be the best option for ensuring and sustaining good well-being. It takes at least two weeks for the body to react to the drastic carbohydrate loss, and occasionally four times as much.

The ketogenic diet usually has unique effects on the body and cells that have benefits beyond what nearly every diet can offer.

Carbohydrate restriction and ketone production mixtures suppress insulin rates, cause autophagy (cell clean-up), boost mitochondrial chemicals' production and effectiveness, minimize inflammation, and burn fat.

PART 2

Intermittent Fasting

Introduction

Whenever fasting is discussed as a cure for obesity and type 2 diabetes, it does obtain the same old eye-rolling reaction. A Hunger? So, is that the solution? Do you want to starve them to death? No. not at all. This is by no way that.

Fasting & Starvation

Fasting is one key aspect that is different from starvation: control. Hunger is the daily abstention from feeding. It is neither intended nor regulated. Starving persons have no clue where and when they can receive their next meal. It occurs in periods of conflict and drought, where there is insufficient food. Fasting, on the other side, is abstaining actively from food for moral, nutritional, or other purposes. Nutrition is freely accessible, but you prefer not to consume it. No matter what the justification for abstaining, a vital point is that fasting is voluntary. Hunger and fasting can never be mistaken, and the words can never be used as interchangeable terms. Fasts and hunger reside in different parts of the world. It's the contrast among running for fun and running when a bear is following you. External forces impose hunger upon them. On the other side, fasting may be performed every time, from a few hours to months on end. You can start a fast at any time of your preference, and you can also end a quick at will. For any cause or no purpose at all, you can begin or end a fast. Fasting doesn't have a traditional period — because it's merely the lack of food, you're fasting when you're not feeding. E.g., the following day, a span of twelve hours or so, you could fast from dinner till breakfast. Fasting can be used as a function of daily life in that way. Fasting is often considered the "old secret" to reducing weight. Why? It's An old method probably dated back thousands of years. Fasting is as sacred as history, far longer than any other eating procedure. But then how is fasting a "secret"? While fasting has been performed for thousands of years, it has mostly been neglected as medical treatment. There are practically no books about it. Very few websites are devoted to fasting. But there is no reference of fasting made in electronic media or print media itself. Just the mere name gathers stares of disbelief. It is a hiding secret in plain view. Why did they do this? Big food corporations have been gradually transforming how we conceive about fasting by the influence of ads. Rather than being a purifying, balanced practice, it is often viewed as something to be hated and at all times prevented. Fasting was incredibly unfortunate for a company; after all, — selling food is hard if people are not going to feed. Fasting has been gradual though ultimately banned. Nutritional authorities also say that only missing a single meal would have severe implications for the well-being.

- You always have to eat breakfast.

- You have had to eat frequently the entire day.

- You must take a snack at bedtime.

- Never have to skip a meal.

Those words appear in books everywhere – on Radio, in the newspaper. Again and again, listening to them produces the impression that they are indeed entirely accurate and objectively verified. The absolute reverse is real. There is simply no connection between regular feeding and good health. Often the officials will want to persuade you that you can't fast since you will be overcome by starvation. It's too hard. This isn't feasible. The reality here is the complete opposite also.

Intermittent Fasting

The expression "intermittent" means "in random intervals." The term fasting is a process for a given period one refrains from a particular task. Basically put Intermittent Fasting (IF) refrains from meals over a certain amount of time.

There are two elements of it

• Fasting: the average time where you keep away from eating

• Feeding period: interval of time at which you may eat.

Myths about Intermittent Fasting

IF is not a miracle weight reduction bomb, you won't lose 10lbs in a week. Even so, you will render regular loss like 1 pound a week.

• IF doesn't say it's the best way of eating for everybody, or the healthiest diet method. IF is a simple diet method that works better for a working person.

• IF is not a must. IF, like any other diet, is just one tool that will help you lose some weight. Look about it as another method to add to the fat-loss toolkit. A variety of different ways to drop weight.

Fasting Benefits

- Improved blood sugar administration

- Lower blood pressure

- Better cardiovascular function

- Less oxidative stress

- Improved metabolic rate during the fast

- Improved fat burning

- Increased appetite control

Chapter 1: Recipes for Fasting Diet

This section of the book contains plenty of ideas for making up your 800 Calories on fast days – do you want three separate meals Or two bigger ones. There are also ways to make a meal a bit 'more significant' with minimum calories inserted, and to allow higher portions for Non-fast time. All calorie counts are proportion.

Berry Parfait

PREP TIME: 15 minutes, plus 30 minutes to chill (optional)

COOK TIME: —

YIELD: 4 servings

INGREDIENTS

- Two tablespoons of 100% pure cocoa powder (optional)
- One cup of heavy whipping cream (at least 45% fat)
- One tablespoon of chia seeds (optional)
- One tablespoon powdered flaxseed (optional)
- 20 blueberries
- 2/3 cup blackberries
- 2/3 cup raspberries
- Six strawberries, very finely sliced
- 12 walnuts, crushed
- 12 almonds, crushed
- Two teaspoons of pure vanilla essence (optional)

- Two teaspoons of cinnamon, for serving (optional)

DIRECTIONS

1. In a cup, put the thick whipped cream and whisk in the chocolate dust and vanilla essence (if using any).

2. Whip your cream till its stiff peaks develop, for about 2 to 3 minutes, using a hand mixer on the medium setting.

3. Optional: Place the container of whipped cream in the refrigerator for up to 30 minutes for a lovely chill on a warm day.

4. Mix in the whipped cream, the nuts, and berries.

5. Mix the soil flaxseed with the chia seeds (if using any) and sprinkle with the cinnamon powder on top, if you wish.

Roasted Cauliflower Rice

PREP TIME: 10 minutes

COOK TIME: 15 minutes

YIELD: Four servings

INGREDIENTS

- One tablespoon Himalayan salt
- Two head cauliflower

DIRECTIONS

1. Preheat your stove to about 200 ° F. Layer a parchment-paper on your baking dish.

2. Split your cauliflower into florets and cut off the roots.

3. Shred the cauliflower by hand or pulse it into a food mixer until it looks like rice.

4. Lay the cauliflower rice onto the baking sheet prepared in the first step and sprinkle with oil.

5. Put the baking tray in the stove and roast, rotating after 5 minutes, for 12 to 15 minutes. Remove before browning with the cauliflower rice.

6. Add any herbs or spices you wish.

Bulletproof Coffee

Throughout recent decades, bulletproof coffee has been quite popular. That may be the case. In fast days, drank once a day to make you stay rested. This is more effective if eaten by the moment you get up and the standard lunch period (although you don't have lunch).

PREP TIME: 2 minutes

COOK TIME: —

YIELD: 2 cups

INGREDIENTS

- 1–2 tablespoons of heavy whipping cream (at least 45% fat)

- 2–3 tablespoons of butter

- 2–3 tablespoons of coconut oil or MCT oil

- Two cups of brewed coffee

DIRECTIONS

1. For the coffee, apply equivalent shares of coconut oil, butter, and sugar.

2. Blend until smooth with an electric blender

Mustard Green Beans

PREP TIME: 10 minutes

COOK TIME: 10 minutes

YIELD: Eight servings

INGREDIENTS

- Two tablespoons of extra-virgin olive oil

- Himalayan salt and ground black pepper

- Two tablespoons of mustard (any kind)

- Two pounds of green beans, trimmed.

DIRECTIONS

1. Fill an average-sized saucepan with just enough water to cover the green beans now over medium-high heat bring it to a boil. Put the beans and boil for around 3 to 4 minutes, until the beans are crisp and juicy. Optionally, you may also steam the beans: Fill a saucepan with water about three-quarters full now add a basket of a steamer on top. At medium-high heat, bring your water to a boil. Now put the beans into the steamer basket and steam for about 5 minutes, until crisp and juicy. Take off the heat.

2. Heat some olive oil over medium heat in a nonstick skillet for about 5 minutes when trying to add the mustard.

3. Place the cooked beans into the mixture of oil and mustard, cook for about 2 minutes, or be well mixed and heated.

4. Take the beans from the skillet, season with salt and pepper, or as required and serve.

Essential Bone Broth

PREP TIME: 10 minutes

COOK TIME: 4 to 48 hours, depending on the kind of bones

YIELD: 6 quarts

INGREDIENTS

- Other herbs or spices (optional)
- Two tablespoons of black peppercorns
- Two tablespoons of Himalayan salt
- Two green bell pepper, roughly chopped
- Two red bell pepper, roughly chopped
- 20 stalks celery, roughly chopped
- Six big carrots, roughly chopped
- Two medium-sized onion, roughly chopped
- Four pounds of animal bones (turkey, chicken, pork, beef, fish, or other)
- Four tablespoons of raw, unfiltered apple cider vinegar

- 12 quarts water

DIRECTIONS

1. Load a saucepan of stock with twelve quarters of cold water.

2. Put some vinegar into the cold water.

3. Put the ribs in the mix of water and vinegar, then let it stay there for about 30 minutes. Prepare the veggies while boiling the bones.

4. Stir in the carrot, onions, bell peppers, celery, salt, pepper, and all other herbs or dried seasoning (if using any).

5. Put it over medium to high heat and heat the water till it is nearly boiling, then cook to low heat. For fish bones, let the stock boil for 4 to 8 hours, for chicken bones boil bones for about 18 to 24 hours; or for beef or pork bones boil for about 24 to 48 h.

6. If it is left to simmer for 30 minutes, incorporate some dried herbs (if using any).

7. Turn off the heat and allow it to cool for around 30 minutes. Then drain out the fat, bones, and vegetables.

8. Place in the fridge for up to 5 days, or freeze in pots, ice cube tubs, or muffin tins, and keep 3 to 4 months in the refrigerator.

Note For more flavor, roast the bones in a 300 ° F stove on a baking tray for 30 minutes until broth is produced.

Homemade Chicken Fingers

PREP TIME: 10 minutes

COOK TIME: 20 to 30 minutes

YIELD: 4 servings

INGREDIENTS

- Four tablespoons of coconut oil

- Two pounds of boneless chicken breasts, trimmed to 1-inch width by 3 inches length

- Two tablespoons of garlic salt (optional)

- Two tablespoons of smoked paprika

- Two tablespoons of freshly ground black pepper

- Two tablespoons of Himalayan salt

- Two cups of crushed pork rinds/cracklings

- Two eggs

- Hot sauce, for serving (optional)

DIRECTIONS

1. Preheat your stove to about 300 ° F. Place aluminum foil on a baking tray.

2. Clean the chicken wings, and pat it to dry.

3. Mix the smashed pork rinds, smoked paprika, pepper, salt, and (if using) some garlic powder into a shallow container. Add the mix into a small sealable box.

4. Beat the eggs in a mid-sized dish. Soak each chicken fingers into the eggs to cover them completely.

5. Now put the chicken fingers covered with egg into the bag with the seasoning mix. Seal and shake the chicken in the bag to cover it with the mix.

6. Put the chicken fingers on your baking dish, then put them in the stove for about 10-15 minutes.

7. Turn the chicken over and cook for another 10 to 15 minutes until it is crispy from both sides and light brown.

8. Take the chicken out of the stove and permit it to cool before served for about 5 minutes.

9. If needed, serve with some hot sauce.

Grain-Free Pancakes

PREP TIME: 10 minutes

COOK TIME: 30 minutes

YIELD: 6 to 8 pancakes (about four servings)

INGREDIENTS

- Ground cinnamon, for topping (optional)

- Two tablespoons of butter or coconut oil, plus more for topping (optional)

- One cup of heavy whipping cream (at least 35% fat), plus more for topping (optional)

- 2/4 teaspoon of Himalayan salt

- One teaspoon of baking soda

- 2/4 cup of coconut flour

- One tablespoon of organic honey or erythritol

- Two teaspoons of vanilla essence

- Four eggs

DIRECTIONS

1. Preheat a grill or pan over low heat.

2. Mix the milk, sugar, vanilla, and honey in one tiny pot.

3. Mix the coconut flour, baking soda, and salt into another medium-sized bowl.

4. Within the dry ingredients, gently mix the wet ingredients.

5. Melt some butter in a skillet.

6. Spill in two or three teaspoons of your batter to shape 3 inches in diameter pancakes. Cook from both sides for 2 to 3 minutes, until lightly browned. Continue for the mixture leftover.

7. Serve the pancakes, with some whipped cream, butter, or cinnamon if desired.

Steak Fajitas

PREP TIME: 10 minutes

COOK TIME: 20 minutes

YIELD: 4 to 6 servings

INGREDIENTS

- Grated cheddar cheese
- Lime wedges
- Pico de gallo

- Guacamole
- Sour cream
- Two pounds skirt steak
- One teaspoon freshly ground black pepper
- Two tablespoons of Himalayan salt
- Large leaves of Boston lettuce (or other lettuce), for serving
- For topping (optional)
- One onion, chopped
- Two yellow bell pepper, thinly sliced
- Two green bell pepper, thinly sliced
- Two red bell pepper, thinly sliced
- Four tablespoons of butter, divided

DIRECTIONS

1. Over moderate heat, prepare a wide skillet. Melt two spoonfuls of butter in the pan.

2. Put the bell peppers and onion, then season it with some salt and pepper. Cook the bell peppers and onion, while occasionally stirring until your peppers are tender, for about 15 to 20 minutes.

3. When almost 10 minutes are remaining for the veggies, warm-up another big skillet over medium heat. Melt the leftover butter two tablespoons into the skillet.

4. When almost 5 minutes are remaining for the veggies, brush your steak with some salt and pepper, and put it with the butter in the skillet. Cook until cooked for about 3 to 5 minutes for each side.

5. Take both the skillets off the fire.

6. Let the steak sit for between 5 and 10 minutes before cutting. Split into required thickness portions.

7. Split the cut up steak and vegetables into 4 to 6 equal pieces and cover each serving in a broadleaf of lettuce. Put the fajita toppings on top and eat!

Mini Frittatas

PREP TIME: 15 minutes

COOK TIME: 20 minutes

YIELD: 12 frittatas (3 to 4 servings)

INGREDIENTS

- 12 slices of bacon
- Two teaspoons of freshly ground black pepper
- Two tablespoons of Himalayan salt
- One cup of grated cheddar cheese (about 2 ounces), plus more for topping(optional)
- One cup of green onions, finely diced
- 2/3 cup of diced green bell pepper
- 2/3 cup of diced red bell pepper
- 24 cherry tomatoes split from the middle
- One cup of chopped spinach
- 12 eggs

DIRECTIONS

1. Preheat your stove up to 300 ° F. Grease coconut oil or butter into a 6-cup muffin tin.

2. Layer your bacon, onions, spinach, green onions, bell peppers, cheese, pepper, and salt in a medium-sized bowl.

3. Roll a bacon strip around the inside wall of each muffins tin. Cut it, then apply it to the egg mix if there is any left.

4. Put in the egg mixture with each muffin tin about three-quarters filled. Topped with cheese (if using any).

5. Put in the stove and cook it for about 20 minutes, or until it's crispy on top.

6. Remove from the oven and allow it to cool before serving for about 10 minutes.

Arugula And Prosciutto Salad

PREP TIME: 10 min

COOK TIME: —

YIELD: Two serving

INGREDIENTS

- Two tablespoons of balsamic vinegar
- Two tablespoons of extra-virgin olive oil

For Your Dressing

- One cup of sliced olives
- One cup of chopped tomato
- 9-12 thin slices of prosciutto
- 3-4 cups arugula, washed

DIRECTIONS

1. Simply throw the tomato, prosciutto, olives, and arugula together in a medium-size container.

2. For making the dressing: Blend olive oil and vinegar together.

3. Put the salad and the sauce together, or serve your dressing on the side.

Simple Homemade Bacon

PREP TIME: 15 minutes, plus 5 to 7 days to cure and 12 hours to chill

COOK TIME: 1½ to 2 hours

YIELD: 4 pounds of bacon

INGREDIENTS

- Any dried herbs and spices (optional)
- Four tablespoons of freshly ground black pepper
- One cup of Himalayan salt
- Four pounds of pork belly

DIRECTIONS

1. Cut the peel with a very sharp blade from the pork belly. Try to keep the skin undamaged, as you cut it in a single piece.

2. Wash the pork belly using some paper towels and pat it to dry.

3. Stir some oil, pepper, and any dried herbs and spices if using any together in a little pot. Add the mixture to your porks belly from both sides.

4. Put the pork belly in an airtight sealed bowl and store it in the refrigerator. It can be stored for up to 5 to 7 days. The earlier you treat it, the better the taste. Turn over the pork belly regularly. (Always wash your hands properly before you do so.)

5. Take out the pork belly from the fridge after the 5 to 7 days are done, and wash off the excess salts, pepper, and all other herbs and spices. Pat it to dry off.

6. Preheat your stove to about 90 ° C (200 ° F).

7. Put a roasting frame in a frying pan. Put the fat side of the pork belly facing up on the frame.

8. Cook until the meat hits a temperature below 150 ° F. This generally takes over an hour and a half to two hours to complete.

9. Take out the pork belly from the stove and allow it to cool for 30 minutes.

10. Roll the meat in waxed paper and store overnight or for 12 hours in the fridge.

11. Cut the meat with a sharp blade down to the required thickness. You can now fry your homemade bacon. Or you may store it in the fridge for up to 5 days, or up to 2 months in the freezer.

Pear And Arugula Salad With Pine Nuts

PREP TIME: 10 minutes

COOK TIME: —

YIELD: Four servings

INGREDIENTS

- One lemon
- One cup pine nuts
- Two pears, thinly sliced
- Eight cups arugula

- Himalayan salt and ground black pepper

- Eight tablespoons of extra-virgin olive oil

DIRECTIONS

1. Simply throw the pear slices, pine nuts, and arugula together in a wide pot.

2. Squeeze some lemon juice over your salad bowl.

3. Pour some olive oil over the salad as well.

4. Season using some salt and pepper, if wanted.

Grain-Free Cauliflower Pizza

PREP TIME: 10 minutes

COOK TIME: 30 to 35 minutes

YIELD: Two 18-inch pizzas (about 6 servings)

INGREDIENTS

- Pizza toppings of your preference
- Two teaspoons of garlic powder
- Two teaspoons of dried oregano
- Two teaspoons of Himalayan salt
- Four large eggs, gently beaten
- Three cups of cauliflower florets (about 2 pounds)

DIRECTIONS

1. Preheat your stove up to 400 ° F. Place a parchment-papered on the baking dish.

2. Pulse the blooming cauliflower in a food blender until finely chopped. Move it to a big bowl.

3. Add the oil, eggs, garlic powder and oregano, together and blend well.

4. Shift the cauliflower mixture to the middle of the pre-prepared baking dish and use your fingers to turn it into a pizza base.

5. Bake for around 20 minutes, or until its light golden.

6. Put the toppings you like, and bake it for another 10 to 15 minutes.

Strawberry And Kale Salad

PREP TIME: 10 minutes

COOK TIME: —

YIELD: Four servings

INGREDIENTS

- Twenty Four strawberries, diced
- Eight cups kale

- Himalayan salt and ground black pepper

- Eight tablespoons of extra-virgin olive oil

- Two tablespoons of balsamic vinegar

- Two cups of walnuts

DIRECTIONS

1. Simply throw the strawberries, walnuts, and kale together in a large mixing bowl.

2. Add some olive oil and vinegar over your salad mix.

3. Top with some salt and pepper, if desired.

Chicken "Breaded" In Pork Rinds

PREP TIME: 15 minutes

COOK TIME: 45 minutes

YIELD: 4 servings

INGREDIENTS

- Four big eggs

- Eight chicken thighs, skin on

- Four teaspoons of smoked paprika

- Four teaspoons of freshly ground pepper

- Two tablespoons of Himalayan salt

- Three cups of pork rinds

DIRECTIONS

1. Preheat your stove to about 375 ° F. Place aluminum foil on your baking tray.

2. Put your pork rinds in a sealed plastic container and crush them using your grip until they look like crumbs of bread. In the pork rinds, Put some salt, smoked paprika, and pepper now shake it until all the ingredients and pork rinds are entirely mixed.

3. Beat the eggs into a tiny bowl.

4. In the beaten eggs, put one of the chicken thighs and leave it in for about 10 seconds.

5. Move the egg-coated chicken thigh to the bag with the crumbled pork rinds and your seasoning. Shake well until the thigh is covered thoroughly, then pick and put on the pre-prepared baking dish.

6. Repeat the above step with all the remaining chicken thighs.

7. In the stove, put the baking tray and bake for 45 minutes or until the chicken turns light golden.

Tomato, Cucumber, And Avocado Salad

PREP TIME: 15 minutes

COOK TIME: —

YIELD: Four servings

INGREDIENTS

- One teaspoon of freshly ground black pepper
- Eight tablespoons of extra-virgin olive oil
- Two tablespoons of balsamic vinegar
- One cup of feta cheese
- Two cups of green olives pitted and halved
- Three cups of cubed avocado (about one large avocado)
- Two cups of halved cherry tomatoes
- Two teaspoons of Himalayan salt
- Four cups diced cucumbers (about one medium cucumber)

DIRECTIONS

1. Simply throw the onions, olives, avocado, and cucumbers together in a medium-sized dish. Sprinkle some feta cheese on top of your salad.

2. Spill the olive oil and the balsamic vinegar over the top and toss.

3. Use salt and pepper to season.

Chicken Drumsticks Wrapped In Bacon

PREP TIME: 5 minutes

COOK TIME: 45 minutes

YIELD: 4 servings

INGREDIENTS

- Eight chicken drumsticks
- Eight slices of bacon
- Three teaspoons of Himalayan salt
- Two teaspoons of freshly ground black pepper

DIRECTIONS

1. Preheat your stove to about 400 ° F. Place some aluminum foil on a baking tray.

2. Place one slice of bacon around each drumstick and make your way from the top section to the bottom of your drumstick. Put on the set baking tray, and add some salt and pepper.

3. Cook for about 45 minutes, or until the bacon looks chewy and delicious.

Avocado Fries

PREP TIME: 15 minutes

COOK TIME: 15 minutes

YIELD: Eight servings

INGREDIENTS

- Juice of one lime

- Four large avocados, cut into ¼-inch-thick slices.

- Four tablespoons of melted coconut oil or butter

- Two eggs

- Dried herbs and spices

- Two tablespoons of Himalayan salt

- Two cups of pork rinds

DIRECTIONS

1. Preheat your stove to about 400 ° F.

2. Put the rinds of pork in a sealed plastic container, and crush it using your hands till they look like crumbs of toast. Combine salt and all other seasoning or herbs that are dried in.

3. Spill some lime juice into a small cup. Whisk your egg in a separate, little pot.

4. Dip every slice of avocado into the lime juice first, then into your whisked eggs. Let it sit in the eggs for about 10 seconds, now flip over to cover the slice's other side.

5. Put the egg-coated avocado slices in the crushed pork rinds within the bag and shake well until the avocado slices are surrounded in a mixture of pork rinds.

6. Put the melted coconut oil into a baking Tray and place the slices of avocado in the tray.

7. Cook for about 15 minutes, or until its light brown.

Chicken Stuffed Bell Peppers

PREP TIME: 10 minutes

COOK TIME: 1 hour 30 minutes

YIELD: Eight servings

INGREDIENTS

- Two tablespoons of butter

- Two clove garlic, minced

- Two small onion, diced

- Two teaspoons of Himalayan salt

- One teaspoon of freshly ground black pepper

- Two teaspoons of smoked paprika

- Two teaspoons of chili powder

- Two cups of grape tomatoes halved

- Two pounds ground chicken

- Six eggs, beaten

- Eight large bell peppers halved

DIRECTIONS

1. Preheat your oven to about 350 ° F. Place a parchment paper on your baking dish.

2. Melt some butter over moderate heat in a pan. Stir in the onion, Chili powder, oil, garlic, paprika, and cinnamon. Sauté for about 5 to 7 minutes.

3. Now mix in the tomatoes and sauté for another 5 to 7 minutes.

4. Add the remaining chicken and cook for about 15 minutes, until golden brown occasionally stirring.

5. Move the cooked meat blend to a mid-sized bowl and add in the eggs gently.

6. Place half cut side up onto the prepared baking dish for each bell pepper. Add your meat and egg mixture into the bell peppers.

7. Put the stuffed peppers in the stove and bake for about 60 minutes until the peppers are mildly soft.

Game Day Wings

PREP TIME: 5 minutes

COOK TIME: About 20 minutes

YIELD: 4 pounds of wings

INGREDIENTS

- Four tablespoons hot sauce (optional)

- Four tablespoons of coconut oil

- Two teaspoons of garlic salt (optional)

- Two tablespoons of smoked paprika

- Two tablespoons of baking powder

- Two tablespoons of freshly ground black pepper

- Two tablespoons of Himalayan salt

- Four pounds of chicken wings

DIRECTIONS

1. Wash and pat dry your chicken wings.

2Add the salt, baking powder, pepper, garlic, and paprika (if using any) in a small bowl.

3. Put your wings in a plastic sealed container, then apply the seasoning mix. Wrap the bag to coat the wings and shake well.

4. Preheat a skillet over medium heat. Melt some coconut oil in the hot pan.

5. Put the wings in the skillet and cover them—Cook for around 10-12 minutes.

6. Switch the wings sides and cook, until golden brown from both sides, for another 10 to 12 minutes.

7. Remove the wings from the heat and allow it to cool for about 5 minutes.

8. Coat the wings, if preferred, with some hot sauce.

Chapter 2: Intermittent Keto Recipes

In common, recipe books are divided into typical groups: breakfast, lunch, dinner, desserts, and snacks. This way, you can consider the recipes set up for comfort. Because keto emphasizes the macronutrients, what is most essential is consuming the correct amounts of food, protein, and carbs. With that in view, feel free to change breakfast for lunch, dinner for dinner, or just breakfast for dinner. Just watch your macros to ensure you don't over-eat all of these.

BREAKFAST

- Cheddar, Spinach & Mushroom Omelet
- Berry Breakfast Shake
- Toad in a Hole
- Blueberry Almond Pancakes
- Cheddar Chive Baked Avocado Eggs
- Bacon, Egg & Cheese Breakfast Muffins.

- Pecan & Coconut' n' Oatmeal

- Boiled Eggs with Spiced Asparagus Soldiers

- Easy Bacon and Egg Muffins

- Baked Salmon and Eggs with Chives

- Porridge with Pistachios and Chia

- Speedy Eggs and Avocado

- Tomato and Basil Omelette

Pecan & Coconut 'N' Oatmeal

This is a nutritious, quick porridge for colder days when you are seeking

a steaming bowl of oatmeal and don't want the carbohydrate explosion.

YIELD: Serves 1

INGREDIENTS

- Four teaspoons of chia seeds

- One cup of coconut or almond milk
- Two tablespoons of coconut flakes
- Two tablespoons of pecans, toasted and chopped
- 2/4 teaspoon pure vanilla extract
- 2/4 teaspoon ground cinnamon
- Four tablespoons of hemp hearts
- Two tablespoons of flax meal
- Four tablespoons of almond flour

DIRECTIONS

1. Mix the flax meal, milk, almond flour, chia seeds, vanilla, hemp core, and cinnamon into a small bowl. Cook over a low flame, continuously stirring for around 5 minutes until softened.

2. Cover with the coconut flakes and pecans, spoon in a pot and eat instantly.

Boiled Eggs with Spiced Asparagus Soldiers

A fantastic sweet, flavorful meal for you.

YIELD: Serves 2

INGREDIENTS

- Eight eggs
- 500g asparagus spears
- large pinch of ground cumin or smoked paprika
- 1 tbsp olive oil

DIRECTIONS

1. Cut or tear off the asparagus' woody edges and blanch the spears for about 3 minutes in a saucepan of hot water. Flush and set it aside.

2. Bring a saucepan of water to a boil. Put your eggs, and boil them for a soft yolk for about 6-7 minutes.

3. Alternatively, fire up a griddle tray on the hob. In the olive oil, dump the asparagus spears and sprinkle some paprika or cumin, add some black pepper and salt. Cook them for about 3-4 minutes on the grill pan, flipping them over a few times till they are soft and lightly sauteed.

4. Serve the eggs using egg cups, with the asparagus griddled to dunk!

Bacon, Egg & Cheese Breakfast "Muffins"

YIELD: Serves 6

INGREDIENTS

- ounces shredded cheddar cheese
- freshly ground black pepper to taste
- Fine sea salt
- 2/4 cup heavy cream
- 16 eggs
- 12 slices of bacon

DIRECTIONS

1. Preheat your stove to about 375ºF. Adequately oil the bottoms and edges of a 6-cup tortilla shell (softened butter serves well for this purpose).

2. Put the bacon to a cold 10 inches skillet, then put the skillet over medium-high heat.

3. Cook the bacon till it's crispy all over, rotating once. Move to a dish layered with paper-towel.

4. Now crumble it into pieces.

5. Whisk together the milk, the eggs, salt, and pepper together in a large bowl.

6. Add an even quantity of cheese and bacon into every cup of the ready tin. Plop a combination of eggs generously over the lining.

7. Bake for about 20 to 25 minutes, till the eggs are golden and puffed up.

Easy Bacon and Egg Muffins

YIELD: Serves 4

INGREDIENTS

- Eight rashers of streaky bacon
- 20g of Parmesan, grated
- Eight eggs

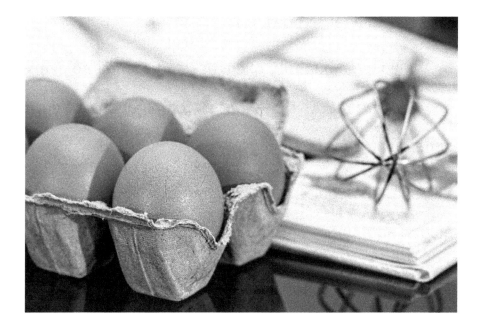

DIRECTIONS

1. Preheat your stove to about 200 ° C/180°C fan/gas point 6.

Very light grease four holes of a silicone or metal muffins tray. Or you may use oven-safe ramekins, also very lightly greased.

2. Break the bacon pieces in two and place them in the muffin holes, making a zigzag shape.

3. Crack an egg in each baked hole.

4. Sprinkle with a freshly ground black pepper and the Parmesan on top. Cook them for a soft yolk for 15 minutes, or a hard yolk for about 20 minutes.

Cheddar Chive Baked Avocado Eggs

YIELD: Serves 2

INGREDIENTS

- Two avocados, cut in half and pitted
- Freshly ground black pepper to taste
- Two teaspoons of fresh chopped chives Sea salt

- Four teaspoons of heavy cream

- ounces cheddar cheese, shredded

- Four eggs

DIRECTIONS

1. Preheat your stove to about 425ºF.

2. In a small dish, add the cheddar cheese, eggs, half of the chives, cream, pepper, and salt. Whisk using a fork until it blends properly.

3. In a shallow rimmed baking dish, place the avocados, cut side up (they must be close, so they don't turn around). Put the egg mixture into the middle of each avocado.

4. Cook for 12 minutes, before the filling, is golden from the top. Serve warm, topped with the chives left over.

Note: Avocado pits differ, and you will need to scrape a little extra avocado from the middle using a spoon to satisfy the filling of the eggs, depending on the thickness.

Baked Salmon and Eggs with Chives

Salmon supplies the brain and body with an excellent omega-3 boost, which helps access the inflammation.

YIELD: Serves 2

INGREDIENTS

- 40g Parmesan, grated
- tbsps of chives, chopped (optional)
- Eight eggs
- A handful of baby spinach or leftover greens, chopped
- 300g smoked salmon

DIRECTIONS

1. Preheat your stove to about 200 ° C/180 ° C and fan/gas point 6. Grease 4 sections of a silicone or metal muffins tray. Conversely, you may use ramekins that are suitable for the stove, greased lightly.

2. Line up the four sections of the tray with the smoked salmon.

3. Bring the spinach into a pot. Using a fork whisk the eggs, Chives, and some black pepper gently in the pot.

4. Split the mixture among the four sections. Sprinkle over the Parmesan, and some more black pepper Now bake for about 15 minutes or until the eggs look ready to consume.

Blueberry Almond Pancakes

Apart from the lack of ingredients, these pancakes vary from the normal in a certain way. When frying, you cover the pan with a lid to guarantee that they heat through in the middle.

YIELD: 10 serving size two pancakes

INGREDIENTS

- Butter to cook the pancakes
- 1 cup blueberries, frozen or fresh
- 2/4 teaspoons of allspice (optional)
- 2/4 teaspoons of sea salt
- Two packet stevia powder
- Two tablespoons of baking powder
- Two tablespoons of flax meal
- 1 cup of almond flour
- 2/4 teaspoon pure vanilla extract

- 2/4 cup almond milk

- Four large eggs

- Eight tablespoons butter

DIRECTIONS

1. Whisk the eggs, vanilla, butter, and almond milk in a tiny pot. Mix in the baking powder, flour, stevia, flaxseed, cinnamon, and allspice until thoroughly mixed. Now fold in your Blueberries.

2. Heat a non-stick pan on medium heat. When a few drops of water start dancing on the pan's surface, it's good to use. Melt some butter in your heated pan.

3. Drop 1/4 cups of flour into the pan and spread it to form a small circle (they 're going to bubble up).

4. Cover the pan with a lid and cook for about 1 to 2 minutes. Before air bubbles emerge on top of the mix and the batter appears a little hot. Switch sides, and cook until crispy and white, maybe for about two more minutes. Serve hot.

Note: Leftover pancakes may be stacked between parchment paper, covered in clear plastic, and held up to 1 week in the refrigerator. Steam them in a 350oF oven right out of the freezer for about 8 to 10 minutes.

Porridge with Pistachios and Chia

With a taste of tropical cardamom, smooth porridge, and the additional value of chia, a superfood rich in minerals, fiber, and protein.

YIELD: Serves 2

INGREDIENTS

- 1 tsp of cardamom seeds
- tbsps of chia seeds
- 600ml milk
- a handful of chopped pistachios
- tbsp rolled oats

DIRECTIONS

1. Put all the ingredients in a saucepan and bring them to a boiling state.

Decrease heat and allow it to boil for another 6-8 minutes, stirring regularly, until your porridge thickens and is fluffy. Toad In A Hole

YIELD: Serves 2

INGREDIENTS

- 2/4 teaspoon sea salt
- Two egg
- 2/4 cup heavy cream
- 12 tablespoons almond milk
- Six tablespoons of arrowroot
- 2/3 cup blanched, fine almond flour
- Eight pork sausages (spicy or sweet)

DIRECTIONS

1. Place an 8 "cast iron skillet on the stove's middle shelf. Preheat your stove to about 400ºF.

2. Stir your sausages into the pan. Cook for about 12 to 15 minutes, often rotating until all are well browned.

3. In a medium-sized dish, mix the arrowroot, almond flour, almond milk, egg butter, and salt. Whisk well until combined thoroughly.

4. After browning the sausages, add the batter into the hot oven. Return the skillet to the oven, and steam for another 20 to 25 minutes until puffed up and golden. Serve straight away.

Speedy Eggs and Avocado

This is for those who complain they have little time to cook breakfast eggs – make them a day before, then arrange them in the morning.

YIELD: Serves 1

INGREDIENTS

- ½ avocado
- Two eggs
- Squeeze of lemon

DIRECTIONS

1. Cook the eggs in a saucepan of boiling water for about 6-7 minutes, then put under cold running water. Peel them out and place them in the refrigerator (if you wash them beforehand).

2. Peel, mortar, and dice the avocado in the morning. Squeeze some lemon juice over it and put it on a tray.

3. The eggs are sliced into pieces. Blend them with the cut avocado and maybe some seasoning.

Berry Breakfast Shake

YIELD: Serves 2

INGREDIENTS

- Two tablespoon MCT oil (optional)
- One teaspoon freshly squeezed lemon juice
- Two tablespoons of almond butter
- 1 cup coconut or almond milk
- 2/4 cup heavy cream
- 2/4 cup frozen mixed berries

DIRECTIONS

1. Put all the ingredients into a food processor. Blend until the mixture is smooth. Serve straight away.

Cheddar, Spinach & Mushroom Omelet

Of course, this is a part of the breakfast section, but omelets are also a perfect afternoon and evening go-to meal, so bear this recipe in mind while preparing your weekly menu.

YIELD: Serves 2

INGREDIENTS

- ounces cheddar cheese, shredded

- 12 eggs, lightly beaten

- Sea salt to taste

- A handful of fresh parsley, chopped

- cups packed baby spinach

- ounces white button mushrooms, sliced

- Four teaspoons extra virgin olive oil

DIRECTIONS

1. Steam up one tablespoon of oil over medium-high heat until shimmering in an 8-inch non-stick skillet. Stir in the mushrooms. Cook, turning the mushrooms a couple of times, for about 3 to 4 minutes, until the mushrooms are translucent. Mix in the spinach and sprinkle some salt on top.

2. Cook for another 1 to 2 minutes, until barely wilted. Now move the vegetables to a pot. Put in the parsley, and set aside.

3. Using the same skillet flame up the remaining tablespoon of oil. Coat the eggs with salt and dump them into the saucepan.

4. Cook till the edges are finished, without damaging the eggs. Raise the egg's undersides while tilting the pan slightly with a rubber spatula so that every uncooked egg will slip underneath and is cooked.

5. Now cover half of the egg with your vegetable mix. Sprinkle some cheese over it.

6. Now fold the plain side of the egg over the veges half to make a half-moon. Cook for another 1 minute. Serve straight away.

Tomato and Basil Omelette

Begin the day off to a good start with this Mediterranean-style excellent Omelet.

YIELD: Serves 1

INGREDIENTS

- 5-6 basil leaves, shredded
- Six cherry tomatoes halved
- 1 tbsp of olive oil
- Four large eggs

DIRECTIONS

1. Beat the eggs using a fork in a pot. Put in some seasoning.

2. Warm the oil in a medium-sized frying pan, and cook your cherry tomato halves for about 2 minutes.

3. Put in the basil and cook for another 20 seconds, then dump in the eggs, Roiling them by a wooden spatula across the pan.

4. When the omelet finishes cooking, remove the edges and fold over. Slide it onto a moist platter to eat when it is partially golden.

LIGHT MEALS

In a perfect world, we will all consume our main meal earlier in the day, adopting the conventional 'Mediterranean' style of cooking, as this means it is least likely to be processed as fat. It doesn't fit everybody, though, so recipes in it segment have been split into 'small' and 'primary' meals, rather than 'lunch' or 'dinner' because you can be creative while you consume them.

The light meals are typically easy and fast to create and usually lower in calories than the main meals. Some function well as brunch as well.

RECIPES:

- BACON, AVOCADO & TURKEY LETTUCE WRAPS

- Hummus in a Hurry

- SPICY SESAME ZOODLES

- Tapenade with Feta

- ITALIAN STUFFED PEPPERS

- WARM SPINACH & ROAST CHICKEN SALAD WITH BACON VINAIGRETTE

Bacon, Avocado & Turkey Lettuce Wraps

Cooking and holding a batch of bacon in the refrigerator allows for quick lunches on a Monday. A simple reheat in a skillet suffices to crisp everything up. Feel free to mix in turkey instead of surplus chicken breast.

YIELD: Serves 4

INGREDIENTS

- Eight slices of cooked bacon

- Two avocados, pitted & sliced

- Two tablespoons of mayonnaise

- Four leaves of curly kale

- Eight slices of turkey

DIRECTIONS

1. Place each kale leaf on a chopping board. Spoon in some mayonnaise. Put two slices of bacon, half of the avocado piece, and two strips of turkey crust on one half of each kale leaf.

2. Roll up beginning with the loaded end. And enjoy.

Hummus in a Hurry

An almost immediate meal that fills the space and tasted fantastic eaten with plenty of crunchy veggies. Don't think about the excessive volume of olive oil – it has advantages for flavor and well-being.

YIELD: Serves 8

INGREDIENTS

- 1 tbsp tahini
- Four garlic cloves, chopped
- tbsps of lemon juice (or more to taste)
- tbsps of extra-virgin olive oil
- 400g tinned chickpeas

DIRECTIONS

1. Drain the chickpeas, and save the water.

2. Mix all the ingredients, apart from 1 tbsp of olive oil.

3. If required to get the correct consistency, put a small quantity of the saved chickpea water. Season the hummus according to your taste, using salt and grounded pepper.

4. Glaze on top with the leftover olive oil and some paprika or cumin seeds, if you like. Serve with some crispy veggie crudités including courgette sticks, celery sticks, cucumber and baby asparagus, cauliflower, or

broccoli florets of which includes very few calories and are a rich source of fiber so that you can consume – nearly full.

Spicy Sesame Zoodles

Cold sesame pasta was once our dream snack. Here we will be swapping in zucchini noodles. Typically the sauces have a flavoring for calming the almond butter's load. But you may include one packet of stevia to the seasoning when you mix it in the pot if you like.

YIELD: Serves 4

INGREDIENTS

- One lime
- 2/4 cup creamy almond butter
- 1 cup shredded red cabbage Handful of fresh cilantro, leaves and

- stems chopped

- Two tablespoons of sesame oil

- Two tablespoons of soy sauce

- One teaspoon of red pepper chili flakes

- Sea salt to taste

- 2/3 cup sliced almonds

- Four scallions, chopped

- Zoodles

DIRECTIONS:

1. The lime is juiced into a large pot.

2. Stir in the dish with soy sauce, almond butter, sesame oil, and chili flakes.

3. Season to salt. Whisk well before combined.

4. Fill the bowl with the cilantro, cabbage, scallions, zoodles, and almonds. Toss to coat thoroughly.

5. Serve right away, or cool before eating.

Tapenade with Feta

The olive paste may have an overly strong and harsh flavor, yet it allows a daintily tangy, creamy spread mixed with feta. Tasty on coin-shaped courgette strips as canapés, or scattered on seeded crackers-or wolfed as a sauce.

YIELD: Serves 4

INGREDIENTS

- tbsps of olive oil
- 100g pitted olives, from a jar or tin, drained
- 100g feta

DIRECTIONS

1. Mix all the ingredients in a tiny cup and a portable blender, leaving several chunky olive pieces.

Italian Stuffed Peppers

YIELD: Serves 4

INGREDIENTS

- Four red bell peppers

- ounces shredded mozzarella

- cup cauliflower Couscous

- One teaspoon dried oregano

- One teaspoon dried basil

- Two garlic cloves, chopped

- 2 cups Slow-Simmered Tomato Sauce

- Freshly ground black pepper

- Sea salt

- 16 ounces of ground beef

- Two tablespoons of extra virgin olive oil

DIRECTIONS

1. Put the oil and flame in a medium pan until shimmering. Put the meat then use a fork to cut up any pieces (little bits of meat you desire). Season with pepper and salt. Cook until brownish. Move to a bowl using a rubber spatula; put down.

2. Put the garlic into the saucepan. Drizzle for about a minute, until aromatic.

3. Add the basil, oregano, and tomato sauce, and bring the beef back into the pan.

4. Mix with pepper and salt. Decrease the heat to low, and cook for about 5 minutes.

5. Preheat your stove to about 375ºF. Retrieve the beef fill from the heat and allow it to cool marginally while the oven is preheating.

6. Stir in the filling Cauliflower Couscous and half of the mozzarella.

7. Chop the heads off the peppered bell and pick the seeds out. And spoon the beef that fills up the peppers. Put the peppers together in an 8-inch loaf pan. Toss over the leftover mozzarella.

8. Bake for about 35 to 40 minutes before the pepper is smooth, and the cheese is golden. Serve warm.

Warm Spinach & Roast Chicken Salad With Bacon Vinaigrette

Most people apply cold bacon to a hot skillet, then hide from the splotches for shelter. The simplest way to avoid it is by adding cold bacon to a cold saucepan. The juices from the foundation for a sweet dressing for what may seem like a rather basic salad. Here the chicken leftover from creating the Bone Broth or the Smoky Butter Roasted Chicken all fit well.

YIELD: Serves 4

INGREDIENTS

- cups packed baby spinach
- Freshly ground black pepper
- Four tablespoons of red wine vinegar
- Four teaspoons of Dijon mustard
- Salt
- Two garlic clove smashed

- cups cubed or shredded cooked chicken

- Eight slices of bacon

DIRECTIONS

1. In a cold 8-inch skillet, put the bacon and put it over medium-high heat. Cook until crispy all over, rotating once. Move to a platter filled with paper towels.

2. Drop the garlic into the same saucepan. Drizzle for about a minute, until aromatic. Lose the cloves. Switch off the flame, swirl in the vinegar and mustard. Mix with pepper and salt, back to medium flame skillet. Add the chicken, and cook for about 1 to 2 minutes until moist.

3. Detach the pan from the heat, stir in the spinach, and split it into four shallow bowls. Savor it right away.

MAIN MEALS

On the whole, these recipes are more significant, and some may take a little longer to plan than the light meals. If you get the main meal at lunchtime or nighttime, it is up to yourself. In fact, the healthier your weight and appetite, the faster you consume your main meal.

RECIPES:

- Spanish Aubergine Stew with Chorizo
- KIMCHI PORK LETTUCE CUPS
- Balsamic Fried Pork Steak with Garlicky White Bean Mash

Spanish Aubergine Stew with Chorizo

A thick, nourishing stew packed with Mediterranean flavors.

YIELD: Serves 4

INGREDIENTS

- 800g tin chopped tomatoes
- Four garlic cloves, sliced

- 200g chorizo, diced

- Two tablespoons of mixed herbs

- Two aubergines, diced

- 240g chestnut mushrooms, sliced

- Two onion, diced

- tbsps of olive oil

DIRECTIONS

1. Sweat your onion in the oil on medium heat for about 4-5 minutes in a casserole dish or a saucepan, then incorporate the eggplant, mushrooms, chorizo, and spices

2. Cook this mixture for about 5 minutes, or until mildly golden, stirring regularly and combining the garlic in the final minute.

3. Stir in the diced tomatoes and half a cup of water (sufficient to release the blend) and let it boil for around 40 minutes, often stirring.

4. Add any steamed greens to serve.

Kimchi Pork Lettuce Cups

This Thai-inspired recipe packs a spice charge. Scrape some pork loading up with a lettuce leaf to feed it, slice it up, and dive deep. You can nix the lettuce for a unique twist and eat the tossed filling with zoodles.

YIELD: Serves 4

INGREDIENTS

- 16 ounces ground pork
- Two garlic clove, chopped fine
- Four teaspoons of extra virgin olive oil
- Two teaspoons of fish sauce (Red Boat fish sauce has no added sugar)
- A handful of fresh cilantro, chopped
- 1 cup kimchi, chopped fine

- Sea salt to taste

- Three teaspoons of soy sauce

- Fresh mint, for garnish

- Two small head Boston lettuce leaves removed, rinsed and patted dry

- Lime wedges, for garnish

DIRECTIONS

1. Heat the oil over medium-high heat in a 10-inch skillet until shimmering. Add the garlic, then sauté for around 1 to 2 minutes until delicately golden.

2. Put the pork split up in some significant bits, using a fork. Stir in the kimchi, coriander, soy sauce, and fish sauce. Season using salt. Decrease the heat to moderate-low. Keep cooking, stirring every few minutes, for up to 7 to 9 minutes, until the pork is fully cooked.

3. In the meantime, organize the leaves on a platter of lettuce. Spoon pouring the fried pork over the leaves of lettuce. Garnish with new mint and the lime wedges. Serve straight away.

Balsamic Fried Pork Steak with Garlicky White Bean Mash

A large steak with a slice of pork mash.

YIELD: Serves 4

INGREDIENTS

For the mash:

- A 2-3cm sprig of fresh rosemary leaves only,
- finely chopped
- Four garlic cloves, diced
- 800g tin cannellini beans (or other white bean),
- water reserved

- tbsp olive oil

- Two small onion, diced

For the steak:

- Two × 300g pork steaks

- 1 tbsp olive oil

- tbsp of balsamic vinegar

DIRECTIONS

1. Warm the olive oil in a saucepan to render the mash and sauté the onion before it is translucent-around 5 minutes. Remove the garlic and cook for 1 minute, then mix in the beans along with their water and gently simmer for about 10 minutes, stirring at times.

2. Put the bean mixture with the rosemary, a good pinch of Maldon oil, and some freshly ground black pepper, and mash it vigorously.

3. Then, over medium heat, put another non-stick frying pan, put the olive oil and fry the pork gently for

about 10-12 minutes, turning it once, until it is brown from both sides and the juices run free.

4. Sprinkle the balsamic vinegar over the steaks and eat them with the mash and Super Simple Greens, a nice slice.

CHAPTER 3: Starting IF Your First 30 Days

The first 30 days of 16:8 aren't drastic, as you may notice. There is no talk here of giving up pasta, potato, or even sweet treats. You will invest the first 30 days making meaningful improvements and delivering fantastic outcomes to support you Motivated to move ahead.

The secret to success, in the long run, lies in how you proceed. You shouldn't rush forward as a beginner, even though you are desperate for results. Initially, the number one excuse people give up is by attempting too hard, too fast. Often, we've been overweight or obese for 5-20 years. It is unrealistic to expect that you will alter long life habits and lack of discipline in a matter of seconds.

Week 1-You're only going to transition to the timeframe of week one.

Tasks

1. Use your ideal feeding period of eight hours. Note that the fasting time has a sleep allocated. Tend to focus the food period on moments you like. It's going to be more challenging not to feed and demonstrate restraint.

2. Don't radically alter the kind of food you consume — this week about getting used to the window of eating.

3. Will not work out. When you're new to fasting workout, appetite would more definitely escalate and make restraint more challenging. Focus just on remaining inside your house.

4. Practice the Monday-Friday 16:8 approach and take the weekend free.

Week 2 – Unless you have managed to adhere to the tasks described in week 1, move to the tasks listed below. We'll discuss sleep next week, and proceed to follow the routine of 16:8 feeding.

Tasks

1. Assessing the eating window last week. Want to alter it? Will, it suits the timetable? If

yes, start using this Monday-Friday time. If no, pick a new window for feeding and replicate week 1.

2. Enforce one of the four strategies for improved sleep presented in this Monday-Friday schedule

3. Enable yourself to walk gently if you have itchy feet! Nonetheless, if you are dealing with the hunger to require maximum modification to your eating schedule, it is advised that you avoid exercise.

4. Again, don't radically alter the kind of food you consume.

Week 3-We 're going to incorporate training next week. You get hanged If you haven't even finished getting any calories down!

Tasks

1. Access the feeding window. Still, working? Does transition need to make you more disciplined? Start with the new window Monday-Friday if the window is correct. If not, pick a new window and then switch back to week 1.

2. Apply necessary HITT instruction according to the ability level. Use the HITT training tips, build a routine to complete two-three days this week. Remember, please check with a qualified doctor before heading into a diet or fitness schedule.

3. Keep on practicing your selected sleep quality tip Week before.

4. Start cutting back on sugar. That task is dependent on the individual. Of course, most people know where to start, but if you need guidance or assistance, please ask your dietitian.

Week 4- You will have the perfect feeding time on the location by week four. When you are still suffering, it is recommended that you contact a community network near you for some more assistance.

Tasks

1. Keep enjoying the slot of your preference Monday-Friday

2. Connect any of the foods for combining magnesium and potassium listed under electrolytes

3. Investigate balanced dessert choices to help you remain calm! Here the key is to include keto sweets because they are rich in fat and weak in carbohydrates. Remember, the fat spikes are less insulin, and will help your body switch to energy fat. Don't buy the drive for "lower fat."

4. Implement a second tip.

5. Continue suppressing sugar

6. Perform 2-4 workouts on HITT

Week 1	MON	TUES	WED	THUR	FRI	SAT	SUN
Morning	KETO	KETO	KETO	KETO	KETO	KETO	KETO
Noon	KETO	KETO	KETO	KETO	KETO	KETO	KETO
Pre 6pm	KETO	KETO	KETO	KETO	KETO	KETO	KETO
Week 2							
Morning	FAST	FAST	FAST	FAST	FAST	FAST	KETO
Noon	KETO	KETO	KETO	KETO	KETO	KETO	KETO
Snack	KETO	KETO	KETO	KETO	KETO	KETO	none
Pre 6pm	KETO	KETO	KETO	KETO	KETO	KETO	KETO
Week 3							
Morning	FAST	FAST	FAST	FAST	FAST	FAST	KETO
Noon	KETO	KETO	KETO	KETO	KETO	KETO	KETO
Snack	KETO	KETO	KETO	KETO	KETO	KETO	none
Pre 6pm	KETO	KETO	KETO	KETO	KETO	KETO	KETO
Week 4							
Morning	FAST	FAST	FAST	FAST	FAST	FAST	KETO
Noon	KETO	KETO	KETO	KETO	KETO	KETO	KETO
Snack	KETO	KETO	KETO	KETO	KETO	KETO	none
Pre 6pm	KETO	KETO	KETO	KETO	KETO	KETO	KETO

3.1 Intermittent fasting tips & tricks

Here's a short rundown of some of IF's main ideas, and what to remember if you decide to test it out.

1. First, consider whether that is right for you. At the same time, the advantages are very cool IF is not for all. Your food and fitness knowledge, and lifestyle, will decide if you are attempting. If you are new to work out and nutrition, then it is recommended that you first learn the basics.

2. Carry on gradually: When you want to seek it, then there is no hurry. Pick one little thing to do, even though it's only a one hour change to daily mealtimes. Give it a shot. See how they go.

3. Instead of being bogged down in the specifics, concentrate on what the solutions have in common. Often, you're fed. Sometimes you don't. Which sort of sums things up.

4. Keep it flexible.

5. Know yourself. Look carefully about your observations. Get savvy. Get going, gather evidence, obtain knowledge, and draw lessons you are using to

direct potential behavior. Choose that which is best for you.

6. Give it time. There's no hurry in there. Mainly because it usually only takes a few weeks to transition to the new system.

7. Check for ups and downs. It's part of everyday life, they happen, and it's component of the method. You'll find out how to get more "fixes" by remaining open-minded and not panicking through the "downs."

8. Talk of what you do want out of IF. Focus on method efficiency and not result.

9. It's as important what you eat as what you don't. We settle started to the food fundamentals. Eat high-quality food at the best days, in the correct quantities. It is enough for certain people to fall into excellent shape—no needed IF.

10. Fit exercise but never overdo it. We highly advocate mixing training with IF to make the best of this. Don't overdo it, please.

Glossary

16/8: A standard method of intermittent fasting (IF) in which you fast every day for 16 hours and consume food in a window of 8 hours. (Eating 10 am-6 pm each day, for instance.)

5/2: A type of intermittent fasting (IF) created by Dr. Michael Mosley, also recognized as the Fast Diet method. This involves five days of daily calorie consumption, and two 500-calorie "fasting" days.

ADF "Alternate Day Fasting: "a type of intermittent fasting (IF) during which usual eating periods are cycled with days of total fasting or extreme calorie restriction.

Autophagy: A cycle of "cleaning up" takes place in the body throughout fasting, through which the body starts to use old damaged proteins in the body to restore development.

Bulletproof Coffee: Bulletproof coffee generally refers to Dave Asprey 's idea of applying fat (such as grass-fed milk, coconut oil, or MCT oil) to one's coffee over a short period of time. Melanie and Gin think this splits the fast. Bulletproof coffee also applies to Dave Asprey's coffee brand and is produced from beans that are verified to be minimal in mold toxins.

"Breaking The Fast": The idea of calorie absorption brings the organism out of the fasted condition.

Delay Don't Deny (3D's): Gin Stephen 's book on the past of her own life, groundbreaking culture, research, and intermittent fasting effectiveness!

Prolonged Fast: Gin and Melanie define prolonged fasts as the ones that last more than a day. We advocate professional care for extended 72 + hour fasting, usually used to manage health problems.

Total Carbs: The number of "productive" carbs in a meal, measured by deducting the fiber grams from a food's overall carb value.

OMAD 'One Meal A Day': a type of extended fasting in which you ingest all of your calories for the day during a single 'meal.' It can merely be one meal (such as breakfast, lunch, or dinner), or it can be a broader meal duration stretching over a food span that may or may not contain 'snacks' and feeding periods. (For example, at "dinner" from 4 pm-8 pm)

Conclusion

16/8 Intermittent fasting (IF) means food only for the next 8-hour period and fast for the subsequent 16 hours. It may facilitate weight loss and increase blood sugar, brain activity, and longevity. During your meal period, maintain a balanced diet and drink calorie-free drinks such as water or unflavored teas and coffee. Until undertaking intermittent fasting, it is essential to consult with the doctor, particularly if you have some existing health problems.

CPSIA information can be obtained
at www.ICGtesting.com
Printed in the USA
LVHW081909230321
682233LV00002B/74